Pocket Picture Guides
Gastroenterology

An **Essential Slide Collection of Gastroenterology**, based on the material in this book, is available. The collection consists of numbered 35mm colour transparencies of each illustration in the book, and each section is accompanied by a slide index for easy reference. The material is presented in an attractive binder, which also contains a copy of the Pocket Picture Guide. The Essential Slide Collection is available from:

Gower Medical Publishing

Middlesex House,
34–42 Cleveland Street,
London W1P 5FB, UK.

101 5th Avenue,
New York, NY. 10003,
USA.

Pocket Picture Guides
Gastroenterology

N. Ian McNeil MA MD MRCP

Lecturer in Medicine, University College London
Honorary Senior Registrar,
University College Hospital
London, UK

J.B. Lippincott Company · Philadelphia
Gower Medical Publishing · London · New York

Distributed in all countries except the USA & Canada by:
Harper & Row International,
10 East 53rd Street,
New York, NY. 10022, USA.

Distributed in the USA & Canada by:
J.B. Lippincott Company,
East Washington Square,
Philadelphia, PA. 19105, USA.

ISBN: 0-397-44561-X (Lippincott/Gower)

Library of Congress Catalog Number: 87–82134

British Library Cataloguing in Publication Data

McNeil, N. Ian
    Gastroenterology.—(Pocket picture
    guides to clinical medicine)
    1. Digestive organs—Diseases
    I. Title   II. Series
    616.3   RC801

Project Editor: Michele Campbell
Design: Ian Spick
Illustration: Pamela Corfield

Printed in Hong Kong by Imago Publishing Ltd.
Set in Palatino and Helvetica by TNR Productions Ltd.,
London.

ACKNOWLEDGEMENTS

I owe much to the assistance and generosity of my colleagues, particularly Dr Martin Sarner and Professor Charles Clark. The radiographs were provided by Drs Edwards, Grant and Walmsley who bore several hours of discussion with patience. The photomicrographs were provided by Dr Jade Chow and Professor Isaacson. To all these, the staff at Gower Medical Publishing and Maureen Furnell and Gillian Brown of the Department of Medicine, I am most grateful. I should also like to thank the following for providing illustrations: Dr DJ Betteridge, University College Hospital, London (Fig.108); Dr P-J Lamey & Mr MAO Lewis, Glasgow Dental Hospital and School (Fig.60); Dr S Lucas, University College Hospital, London (Figs.95 & 97); Professor CF McCarthy, Regional Hospital, Galway (Fig.45); Dr PH McKee, St Thomas's Hospital Medical School, London (Fig.49); Dr PH McKee & Dr CDM Fletcher, St Thomas's Hospital Medical School, London (Fig.94); Dr K Matthewson, University College Hospital, London (Figs.24, 27, 29 & 39); Dr R Miller, University College Hospital, London (Fig.78); Dr P Salmon, Middlesex Hospital, London (Figs.62, 110, 115, 118, 123, 125, 126 & 150); Dr DE Sharvill, formerly of the William Harvey Hospital, Ashford, Kent (Figs.38, 43 & 47); Mr DJ Spalton, St Thomas's Hospital, London (Fig.150); Dr P Swain, St George's Hospital, London (Fig.26); from the slide collection of Guido Tytgat, MD (Figs.21, 68, 69, 85, 86, 99, 100 & 142).

N.I. NcNeil,
London

PREFACE

My aim in preparing this book has been to provide a
visual approach to diagnosing gastrointestinal disease.
For several years great technical advances have been
made in the investigations used and their features
have been included as well as those clinical
appearances that lead to a diagnosis. Common and
important diseases have been selected in the most
part. Inevitably, some conditions will produce a
disproportionate number of illustrations so this
volume should be read, as intended, in conjunction
with one of the many standard textbooks of
gastrointestinal and liver disease.

N.I. McNeil,
London

CONTENTS

Acknowledgements   v

Preface   vi

Oesophageal Disorders   1

Disorders of the Stomach and Duodenum   11

Disorders of the Small Intestine   22

Inflammatory Bowel Disease   27

Disorders of the Large Intestine   43

Pancreatic and Biliary Disorders   54

Disorders of the Liver   68

Index   83

OESOPHAGEAL DISORDERS

The principal symptoms produced by oesophageal disease are pain and dysphagia. Heartburn is the commonest pain, being a retrosternal burning radiating to the neck: bitter fluid may be tasted during an attack which is typically meal or posture related. Spasm is a severe, tight, central chest pain which also occurs most often after meals. It can be extremely difficult to separate from ischaemic cardiac pain. Least frequent is odynophagia, the pain produced by food or liquid touching inflamed mucosa caused, for example, by reflux oesophagitis or monilia. Dysphagia (difficulty in swallowing) may be caused by many pharyngeal and oesophageal conditions. As physical signs are few or absent, diagnosis depends on an accurate history and appropriate investigations. Those most commonly employed are barium swallows and endoscopy. Tests for acid reflux by pH recording and manometry for motility disorders are less frequently needed.

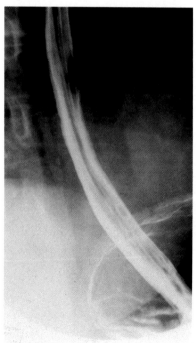

Fig.1 Normal barium swallow. Several identical pictures were obtained during this normal examination. A few air bubbles are also present since most people swallow some air with liquids and solids. Pleating of the mucosa running along the lumen can be seen. As well as obtaining static pictures, the radiologist should also see that normal swallowing occurs on screening.

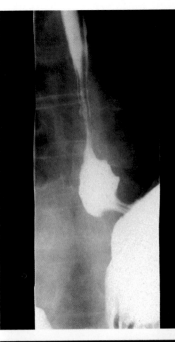

Fig.2 Sliding hiatus hernia. This is the most frequently obtained view of a sliding hiatus hernia on a barium study. The barium filled stomach is seen (lower right) with an extension above the diaphragm, the hiatus hernia. Symptoms, if any, from this common finding will be heartburn due to reflux oesophagitis and acid regurgitation.

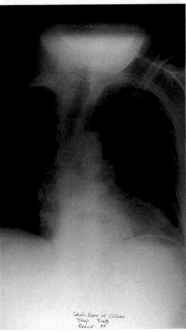

Fig.3 Hiatus hernia on chest X-ray. A fluid level behind the heart is almost invariably produced by a hiatus hernia. This patient had severe chest pain which could not be distinguished from ischaemic cardiac pain. However a normal ECG and history of indigestion led to a barium meal which showed a rolling hiatus hernia (Fig.4).

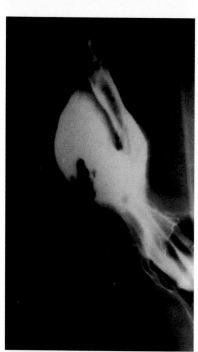

Fig.4 Rolling hiatus hernia. This lateral view shows a rolling or para-oesophageal hiatus hernia behind the oesophagus. The patient was thought to be at risk of torsion of the stomach because of the severe pain she had experienced and surgical repair of the hernia was undertaken as an emergency.

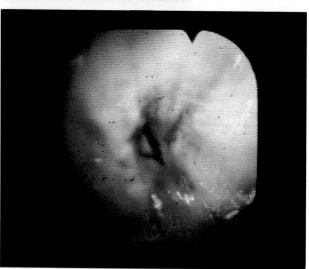

Fig.5 Reflux oesophagitis. Blood is present in this endoscopic view because the inflammation is friable. The red streaks radiating up the mucosa are those typically seen in moderately severe oesophagitis.

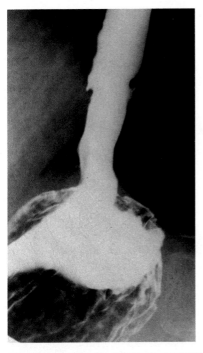

Fig.6 Oesophageal ulceration. Ulceration is present several centimetres proximal to the stomach. The diagnosis was confirmed by endoscopic examination which showed a crater with surrounding inflammation. The symptoms were retrosternal pain on swallowing (odynophagia) and slight dysphagia. Treatment for reflux oesophagitis provided an effective cure. Some drugs, including emepronium bromide, aspirin and slow-release potassium have been found to cause oesophageal ulceration.

	Benign strictures	**Malignant strictures**
Symptoms	preceding heartburn and regurgitation, variable dysphagia	no heartburn, progressive dysphagia
Radiology	hiatus hernia and reflux, ± ulceration, short smooth stricture, proximal dilatation if long history	long irregular stricture with shouldering, proximal dilatation rare
Endoscopy	inflamed oesophagus, sudden narrowing	normal mucosa to stricture, irregular heaped-up mucosa due to underlying tumour and possibly views of malignant tissue

Fig.7 A comparison of benign and malignant oesophageal strictures. Both occur with increased frequency in the elderly. Endoscopy with biopsy and brush cytology is most important in confirming the clinical diagnosis. Treatment depends on the nature of the stricture.

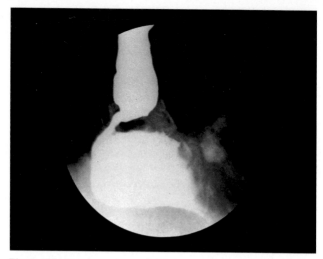

Fig.8 Benign oesophageal stricture: radiology. A peptic stricture is visible between a slightly dilated oesophagus and a sliding hiatus hernia. Endoscopic dilatation was successful in relieving the symptoms in this elderly lady. Repeated dilatations are often necessary as the stricture may recur.

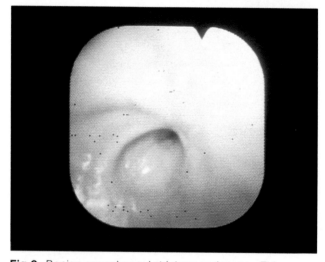

Fig.9 Benign oesophageal stricture: endoscopy. This stricture in an elderly lady measured 5mm in diameter yet was not associated with significant symptoms. The mucosa can be seen tapering smoothly into the stricture. It is likely that this patient's diet had adapted gradually with the tightening of the stricture, preventing the complaint of dysphagia.

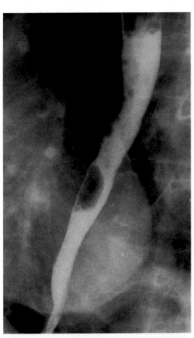

Fig.10 Caustic oesophageal stricture. A progressive narrowing of the oesophageal lumen is seen below the large bubble, extending smoothly over several centimetres. This was caused by the accidental swallowing of lye (potassium hydroxide solution). The patient was accustomed to dilating the stricture with a mercury bougie at home when dysphagia became troublesome.

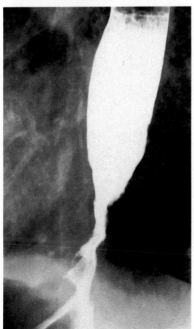

Fig.11 Early oesophageal carcinoma. A barium swallow is an important first investigation of dysphagia. Adenocarcinoma involving the gastro-oesophageal junction can be a difficult diagnosis to make. An irregular lower oesophageal stricture is the most common finding but it can be mistaken both radiologically and endoscopically for reflux oesophagitis. The malignant nature of this stricture was not recognised until histology and cytology had been obtained.

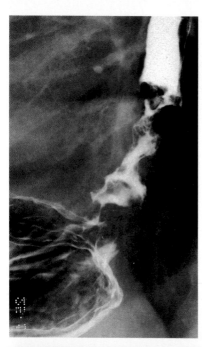

Fig.12 Advanced oesophageal carcinoma. This is a long squamous carcinoma of the middle and lower thirds with shouldering at its upper limit. Oesophageal carcinoma is most commonly found at this site and the patients are usually men. This patient had severe dysphagia and the tumour was sufficiently large to produce anaemia.

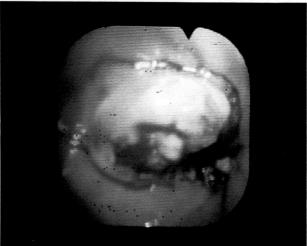

Fig.13 Oesophageal carcinoma. Bulging, friable nodules of tumour are present in the lumen. Longitudinal extension is typical and the mucosa over these nodules may be normal so that small biopsies may miss the underlying neoplasm. The cytology brush is very useful as it can obtain malignant cells from the exposed carcinoma within the stricture.

7

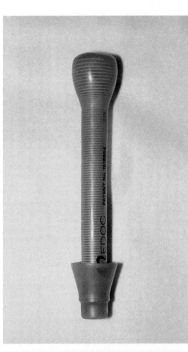

Fig.14 Celestin tube. This tube has an internal diameter of 1–1.5cm and can be placed across an oesophageal stricture to enable the resumption of swallowing. It is generally used for the palliation of malignant strictures. Celestin tubes can be placed using an endoscopic technique after the stricture has been dilated, or at surgery when they are pulled down via a gastrotomy.

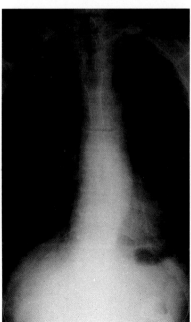

Fig.15 Celestin tube *in situ*. The stiffening rings of a celestin tube can be seen in outline against the dorsal spine. Blockages do occur but can be cleared endoscopically. Patients are recommended to chew any food very carefully and to swallow with aerated water to minimise the risk of blockage.

8

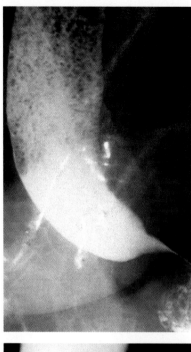

Fig.16 Achalasia. This dilated oesophagus contains food residue above the barium. Little peristalsis was observed on screening. The oesophagus tapers in a typical manner at the lower oesophageal sphincter. Administration of amyl nitrate or nifedipine may improve swallowing temporarily but forcible rupture or a myotomy with anti-reflux procedure are usually needed for significant, maintained benefit.

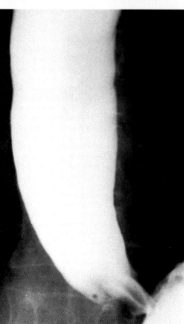

Fig.17 Scleroderma. Atrophy and fibrosis of the muscle of the lower two thirds of the oesophagus in scleroderma leads to progressive dilatation. Dysphagia is a common symptom. Gastro-oesophageal reflux and the impaired peristaltic clearance of acid from the oesophagus may produce severe oesophagitis and benign stricture.

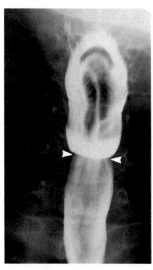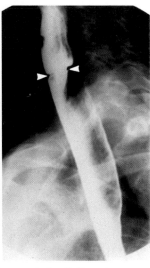

Fig.18 Oesophageal web. Anteroposterior (left) and lateral (right) views confirm the circumferential nature of an upper oesophageal web (arrowed). Intermittent dysphagia is the usual indication for the barium swallow that finds the web. Webs can be associated with koilonychia (sideropaenic dysphagia) and those who have had a web show an increased incidence of upper oesophageal carcinoma.

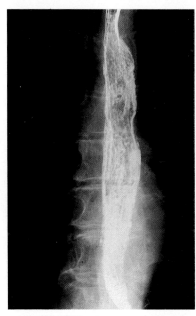

Fig.19 Monilial oesophagitis. The ragged pattern of the mucosa is very suggestive of monilia. If white plaques are seen in the pharynx no further investigation is needed unless the patient fails to respond to appropriate treatment. In the elderly or seriously ill patient monilial oesophagitis can be a cause of malaise and weight loss but little pain or dysphagia is present.

DISORDERS OF THE STOMACH AND DUODENUM

Indigestion, a burning epigastric pain, is the cardinal symptom of diseases of the stomach and duodenum. In peptic ulceration, the relationship of the pain to meals and how it is relieved afford valuable clues to the diagnosis. Peptic ulceration commonly follows a course of remission and relapse over many years. Vomiting and weight loss suggest malignant disease or pyloric obstruction. As a first investigation endoscopy is being used increasingly often, the barium meal becoming less frequent. Gastric ulceration on a barium meal is an indication for endoscopy so that examination of the ulcer and the collection of biopsies to exclude malignancy can be undertaken. The medical management of peptic ulcers has changed dramatically over the past decade with the introduction of a series of proven therapeutic agents. Surgery is becoming less common and may decrease further as new drug treatments continue to be introduced.

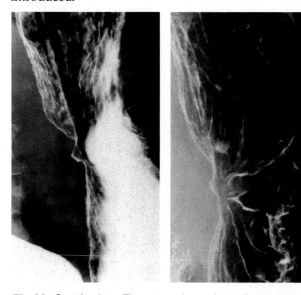

Fig.20 Gastric ulcer. These two views of gastric ulcers on the mid-lesser curve show how a benign ulcer generally protrudes from the line of the surrounding mucosa. The case on the right is in the process of healing; radiating folds produced by the contraction of the associated fibrous tissue are evident.

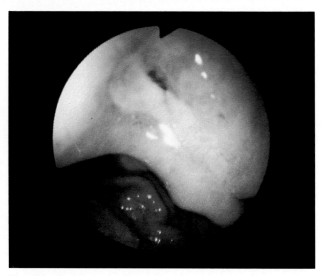

Fig. 21 Gastric ulcer. The white slough of an ulcer is seen on the lesser curve. It appears benign, without the heaped or rolled edges of a malignant ulcer. Biopsies and cytological samples should be taken at endoscopy to confirm its nature.

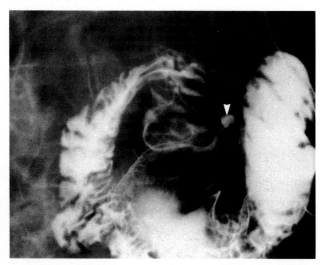

Fig. 22 Duodenal ulcer. A characteristic pool of barium (arrowed) with radiating folds is seen *en face*. Duodenal ulceration is an illness with recurrent episodes of pain lasting for a few weeks followed by months without pain. The ulcers usually heal spontaneously although medical treatment speeds this process and increases the numbers that heal.

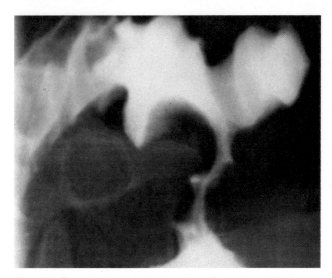

Fig. 23 Chronic duodenal ulceration. The antrum lies just below the lower margin of the picture. The duodenum is distorted and puckered, the result of chronic duodenal ulceration, although no ulcer crater could be demonstrated on this occasion.

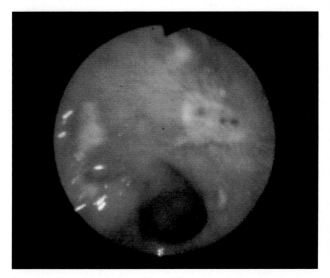

Fig. 24 Duodenal ulcer. The white base of the ulcer contains ulcer slough with underlying granulation tissue. The surrounding mucosa is inflamed and erythematous. Paired or 'kissing' ulcers are present on opposite walls of the duodenum.

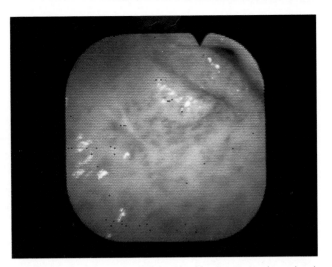

Fig. 25 Duodenal scar and duodenitis. As acute ulcers heal they regress until only a scar remains as visible evidence of their presence. The red spots on the surrounding mucosa indicate persisting inflammation with little ulceration, the characteristic endoscopic appearance of duodenitis. Further healing of the scar distorts the duodenum, producing the pouches seen beyond the scar.

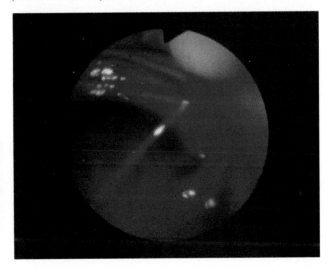

Fig. 26 Bleeding gastric ulcer. A jet of arterial blood can be seen crossing the field of view from a gastric ulcer. Frank arterial bleeding is fortunately uncommon and early surgery is generally indicated as the only satisfactory way of achieving haemostasis.

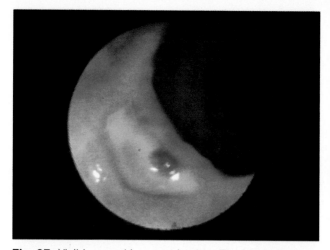

Fig. 27 Visible vessel in a gastric ulcer. The ulcer adjacent to the pylorus contains a swelling which is an exposed and ruptured artery. A visible vessel is an important adverse prognostic factor in predicting the likelihood of rebleeding. Although biopsy and cytology specimens will be required, it is prudent to wait until several days after the bleeding has stopped.

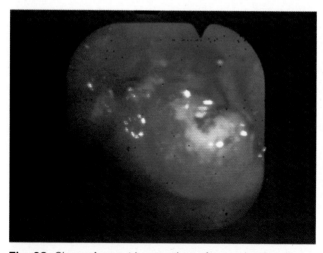

Fig. 28 Signs of recent haemorrhage from a duodenal ulcer. Peptic ulceration is the commonest cause of haematemesis and melaena. The appearance of this ulcer with haemorrhage and altered blood in the ulcer base confirms that it must have been the source of a recent haemorrhage, even if other lesions (such as oesophageal varices) that could have bled had been present.

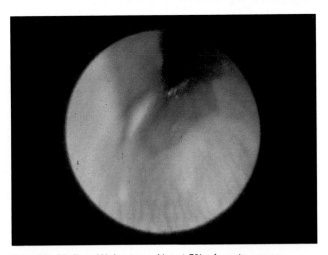

Fig. 29 Mallory-Weiss tear. About 5% of acute upper gastrointestinal bleeds arise from a Mallory-Weiss tear which is produced by the strain of retching and vomiting. Classically, blood is not seen on the initial vomit. Endoscopically, a linear break in the mucosa is seen passing from paler oesophageal mucosa to the pink gastric mucosa beyond. In general no active treatment is required.

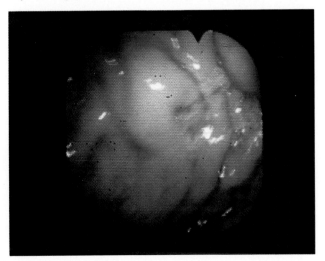

Fig. 30 Gastric erosions. Erosive gastritis is a common source of gastrointestinal bleeding. Recognised causes include alcohol, aspirin, severe stress and infection. It is fortunate that bleeding generally stops spontaneously as endoscopic treatment can be very difficult and surgery may require an extensive gastrectomy.

16

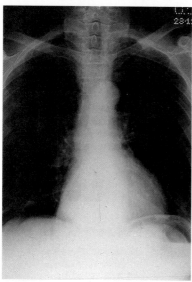

Fig. 31 Perforated peptic ulcer. The sudden onset of severe upper abdominal pain spreading to involve all the abdomen and possibly the shoulders is the usual symptom of a perforated ulcer. Examination reveals considerable rigidity and free gas outlining the diaphragm from below is generally seen on a chest X-ray. The treatment is surgical in all who are able to stand an operation.

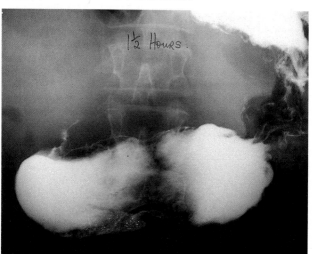

Fig. 32 Pyloric stenosis. This photograph, taken 90 minutes after the start of a barium meal, shows a greatly distended stomach and no passage of barium into the duodenum. A thin line of barium is seen in the region of the pylorus. Pyloric stenoses can complicate duodenal ulceration and gastric carcinoma. Copious vomiting, weight loss and metabolic disturbance result. Endoscopy to ascertain the cause should be undertaken after a prolonged fast with adequate intravenous fluids and, if necessary, gastric lavage to remove food residue.

17

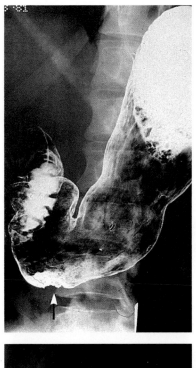

Fig. 33 Carcinoma of the stomach. This, one of several identical views that confirmed the consistency of the appearance, shows an irregular deformity (arrowed) of the greater curve at the junction of the antrum and body of the stomach. The lesion can be seen to protrude into the lumen from the anticipated line of the mucosa. Endoscopy with biopsy confirmed the diagnosis of carcinoma.

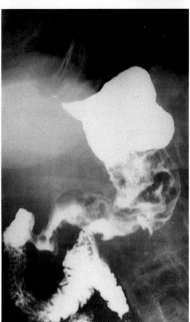

Fig. 34 Gastric carcinoma. Advanced carcinoma has produced a contracted stomach with most of the body and antrum appearing irregular and rigid. Polypoid masses of tumour can be seen. The fundus seems to be spared.

18

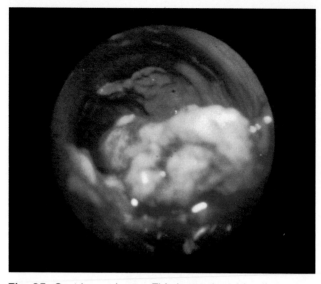

Fig. 35 Gastric carcinoma. This heaped-up, bleeding gastric cancer is at an advanced stage. Endoscopy can assist the surgeon by confirming the diagnosis histologically and by estimating the separation of the tumour, if any, from the pylorus and, more importantly, from the cardia.

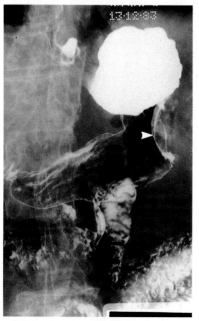

Fig. 36 Leiomyoma of the stomach. The smooth, rounded filling defect (arrowed) on the greater curve of the stomach is produced by a leiomyoma. Gastric folds are often seen to be displaced by this benign tumour. No apical ulcer is visible on this example.

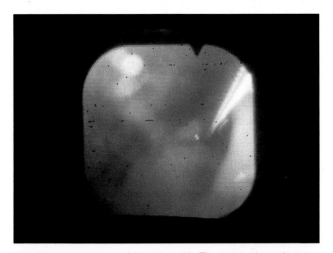

Fig. 37 Leiomyoma of the stomach. These tumours show as bulges beneath the gastric mucosa. Biopsy forceps are pointing to the ulcerating pit at the centre of the tumour which is a source of bleeding, the most common symptom in those cases that are symptomatic. Leiomyomas should be removed surgically if they are symptomatic or if there is any doubt about their innocence.

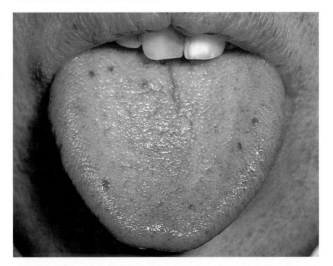

Fig. 38 Hereditary haemorrhagic telangiectasia. Cherry-red vascular anomalies are seen on the lips and tongue. They may also be seen to a lesser extent on the hands and other skin surfaces. As well as producing chronic gastrointestinal bleeding, telangiectasia in the nasopharynx can lead to severe epistaxis. Lesions are rarely found before middle age.

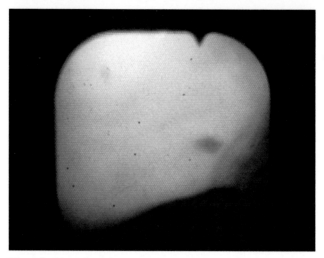

Fig. 39 Hereditary haemorrhagic telangiectasia. This is a gastric telangiectasis. Patients with the syndrome are likely to have many scattered over the mucosa; more than one may be bleeding. In some centres endoscopic therapy with diathermy or lasers has largely replaced surgery as a method of containing blood loss.

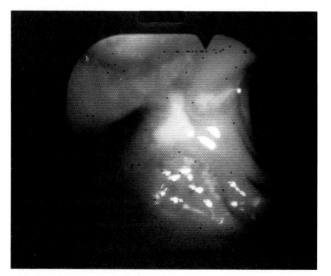

Fig. 40 Stomal ulcer. Recurrent ulceration after surgery occurs in up to 16% of patients depending on the type of operation performed. This illustration shows a white ulcer crater in the jejunum bridging the afferent and efferent loops of a gastroenterostomy.

DISORDERS OF THE SMALL INTESTINE

Malabsorption is the usual consequence of small intestinal disease. Multiple deficiencies of nutrients when intake is normal should lead to a series of investigations for malabsorption. The history is often not of significance for a specific diagnosis but a barium meal follow-through may disclose many of the causes of malabsorption. Jejunal biopsy with aspiration of intestinal contents for microbiology is likely to follow. Thereafter specific investigations should be undertaken as appropriate. In most cases treatment is succeeded by a dramatic improvement in the patient's wellbeing and rapid correction of the nutrient deficiencies. Tumours in the small intestine are rare but are an important cause of obscure chronic intestinal bleeding, often needing angiography to reveal them.

Anatomical (postoperative)
post-gastrectomy
jejunal resection

Pancreatic
chronic pancreatitis
pancreatic carcinoma
cystic fibrosis

Biliary
obstructive jaundice
ileal resection

Mucosal
coeliac disease
Whipple's disease
alactasia

Infection
small bowel bacterial overgrowth
blind loop syndrome
tropical sprue

Infestation
giardiasis
intestinal worms

Inflammatory
Crohn's disease

Others
irradiation
ischaemia
thyrotoxicosis
drugs e.g. neomycin

Fig. 41 Causes of malabsorption. This list is far from exhaustive and is drawn up to outline the commoner or more important causes, many of which act by more than one mechanism. Considering the cause in this way leads to a plan of investigation for patients with established malabsorption.

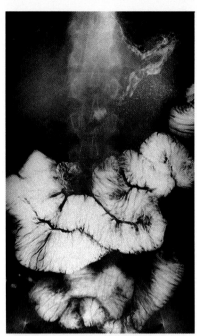

Fig. 42 Malabsorption pattern on barium follow-through. Malabsorption is indicated by widening of the jejunal loops to a maximum of 5.4 cm (normal <3 cm). The valvulae conniventes across the loops are thickened. Some dilution of the column of barium has occurred with flocculation; the pattern is non-specific. In this instance coeliac disease was established by biopsy.

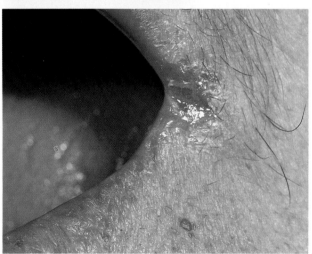

Fig. 43 Angular stomatitis. A feature of iron deficiency as well as vitamin deficiencies (particularly B_6 and B_{12}). There is associated fissuring of the lips in many patients. The lesions settle as treatment is established. Patients with iron deficiency of a long duration may also present with koilonychia (spoon-shaped nails).

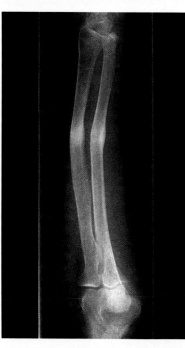

Fig. 44 Osteo-malacia. Pseudo-fractures (Looser's zones) are evident in the bones of the forearm. These indicate osteomalacia which can result from malabsorption of calcium and vitamin D or from gastrectomy for peptic ulceration. The pseudofractures heal after a few months treatment with calcium and vitamin D and the radiographs revert to normal.

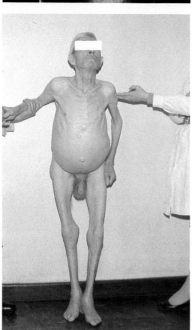

Fig. 45 Coeliac disease. This man is weak and wasted, but is not oedematous. His abdomen is very distended and he is prematurely grey. Nutritional supplements and a gluten-free diet will induce a rapid improvement in his condition but it will take many months to restore him to his correct strength and size.

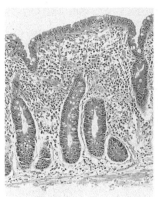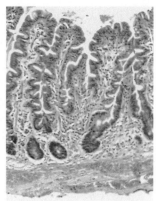

Fig. 46 Coeliac disease. The response to a gluten-free diet. Prior to treatment (left) the mucosa is oedematous and the villi so thickened that they have lost their shape. There is a dense inflammatory cell infiltrate and numerous lymphocytes are present in the surface epithelium. The crypts that extend down to the muscularis mucosa are enlarged and contain numerous mitoses. After treatment (right) the villi appear finger-like and contain few inflammatory cells. The crypts are much smaller and there are very few intraepithelial lymphocytes. Electron microscopy will demonstrate the return of the brush border. H & E stains.

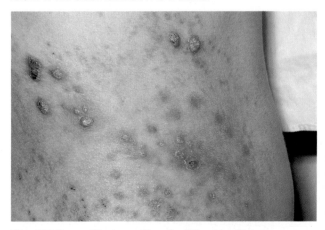

Fig. 47 Dermatitis herpetiformis. This skin disease presents with itchy plaques that blister. Almost all patients have small intestinal changes similar to coeliac disease and malabsorption can be demonstrated in some. Dapsone is used to control the cutaneous lesions. On a gluten-free diet the intestinal mucosa returns to normal and the dose of dapsone needed is much reduced or may no longer be required.

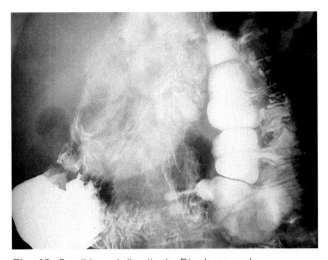

Fig. 48 Small bowel diverticula. Diarrhoea and malabsorption due to small bowel bacterial overgrowth (blind loop syndrome) are thought to take a prolonged period to develop after diverticula have formed in the jejunum of the elderly. The size and number of the diverticula vary considerably; in this case they are particularly large and numerous. Although diagnosis is best confirmed by culturing the contents of the small intestine, many patients are frail and elderly so the clinical response and improvement in a breath hydrogen study to a therapeutic trial of antibiotics is often tried first.

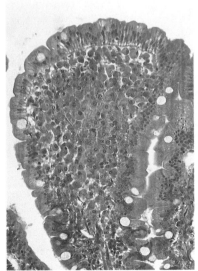

Fig. 49 Whipple's disease. The PAS-positive macrophages packing the lamina propria and distorting the normal architecture are characteristic. Though rare, this illness is of interest as it is due to intracellular bacteria. Involvement of the heart, lungs and brain may occur. The malabsorption and, more slowly, the histology resolve after prolonged antibiotic treatment. PAS stain.

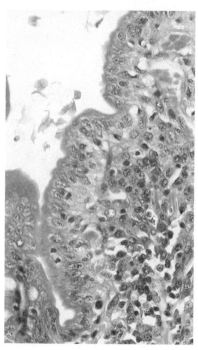

Fig. 50 Giardiasis. These jejunal villi are abnormal with a considerable excess of plasma cells present. The disc-shaped trophozooites of *Giardia lamblia* can be seen in the lumen. Many people have asymptomatic infections but diarrhoea, pain and nausea are frequently experienced and malabsorption may be detected. Metronidazole, 2g for each of three days, is the usual treatment. H & E stain.

INFLAMMATORY BOWEL DISEASE

Inflammatory bowel disease may be less frequent in the population than peptic ulceration and functional disorders but the toll of the illness in relapse and in continuing symptoms means that considerable time and attention are needed from the gastroenterologist. Almost all patients can be categorised on clinical, radiological and histological grounds into ulcerative proctocolitis or Crohn's disease and this has implications for prognosis and treatment. The incidence of both is probably still increasing and despite much attention, the aetiology is unknown. There are many extra-intestinal manifestations, only some of which respond to treatment of the disease or excisional surgery. Advances in treatment are slowly being made as a greater understanding of the diseases and their current therapies is gained. Close cooperation between physician and surgeon is an important aspect of the management of those patients with more difficult inflammatory bowel disease.

	Ulcerative colitis	Crohn's colitis
Symptoms:		
diarrhoea	in many	very frequent
bleeding	very frequent	occurs
mucus	frequent	occurs
pain	variable	frequent
Anal lesions	occasional	common
Sigmoidoscopic appearance	inflamed mucosa with oedema, contact bleeding, mucopus, ulceration	inflamed or normal mucosa, ± aphthous ulcers
Histology	mucosal inflammation, goblet cell depletion, crypt abscess, superficial ulceration	transmural inflammation, deep ulceration and fissuring, granulomas, patchy involvement
Radiology	rectal involvement with variable proximal extension, superficial ulceration with collar stud ulcers in severe cases, pseudopolyps	skip lesions, rectal sparing, ileal disease, rose thorn or aphthous ulceration, fistulae and strictures, cobblestone mucosa, asymmetrical involvement

Fig. 51 Ulcerative and Crohn's colitis compared. The most useful features for separating the two conditions are given. Unfortunately, many are not confined to either condition and may occasionally be seen in both diseases. In up to 5% of patients with acute colitis it proves impossible to reach a final conclusion (indeterminate colitis).

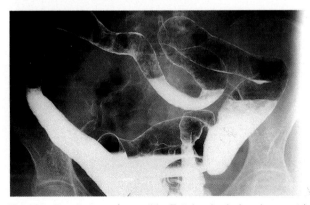

Fig. 52 Total ulcerative colitis. Total colonic involvement in ulcerative colitis is shown by the fine ulceration and the contracted, tubular colon. No haustra are visible. The rectum is obscured by barium that has passed an incompetent ileocaecal valve and filled the ileum.

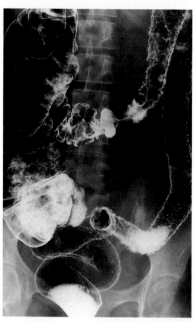

Fig. 53 Ulcerative colitis: extensive active disease. Inflammation extends continuously from the rectum to the mid-transverse colon. The inflammation in the rectum is of the severity most commonly seen on barium studies, but in the descending colon the disease is more severe with abscesses and inflammation undermining the mucosa. Left-sided colitis and, in some cases, proctitis are often complicated by proximal faecal retention, as in this example.

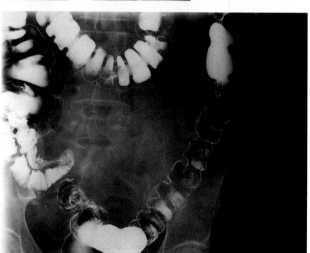

Fig. 54 Inactive left-sided ulcerative colitis. Inactive but long-standing ulcerative colitis is manifest by numerous pseudopolyps, seen here in the left colon. They represent mucosal remnants not destroyed in one of the acute attacks which the patient had previously suffered. There is no ulceration of the colon between the pseudopolyps.

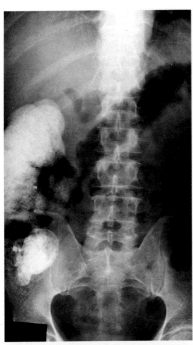

Fig. 55 Mucosal oedema in inflammatory bowel disease. This patient has had a recent barium study. The transverse colon and particularly the splenic flexure show an abnormal outline with bulging, oedematous mucosa left as islands by the surrounding inflammation. These will become the pseudopolyps of long-standing ulcerative colitis.

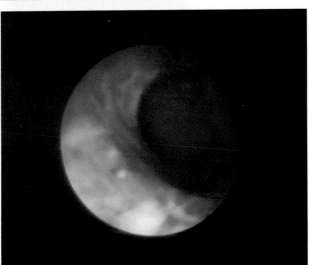

Fig. 56 Acute ulcerative colitis. In this endoscopic view there is a featureless mucosa with both sheet and pinpoint ulceration. No blood vessels are visible. The lumen is tubular.

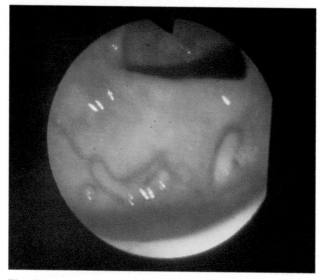

Fig. 57 Inactive ulcerative colitis. This endoscopic view shows the pale mucosa of inactive ulcerative colitis. None of the pseudopolyps is red or inflamed. A single haustral fold is visible and blood vessels are just discernable in the mucosa.

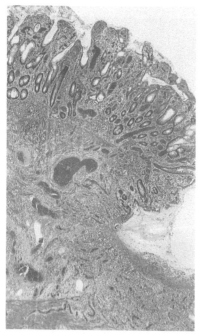

Fig. 58 Histology of ulcerative colitis. Severely inflamed with considerable engorgement of the blood vessels, this island of mucosa is adjacent to a large flat ulcer in the submucosa. Many of the glands are branched, suggesting regeneration and only a few crypt abscesses remain. If recovery continues, this remnant of mucosa is likely to become a pseudopolyp. H & E stain.

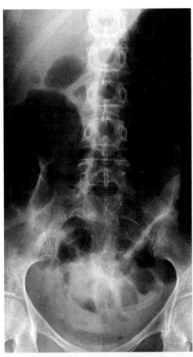

Fig. 59 Toxic dilatation of the colon. This complication of a severe attack of ulcerative colitis is only rarely seen in Crohn's colitis. The appearance of a greatly dilated colon with a reduced haustral pattern in the context of a severe attack is generally considered an indication for emergency colectomy as 20-40% subsequently perforate. Even if the patient should initially appear to respond to medical management, the colitis never fully remits and colectomy is the fate of the majority.

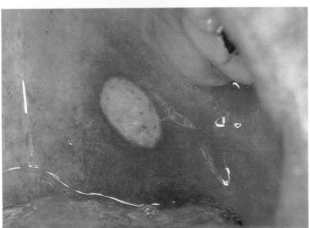

Fig. 60 Mouth ulcers. Aphthous ulcers are common, taking one to two weeks to heal. The visible features of a yellowish ulcer with surrounding redness are the same as those of any ulcer, for example gastric or colonic. They occur with increased frequency in inflammatory bowel disease and coeliac disease.

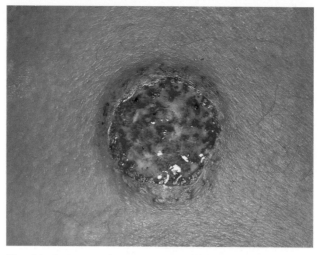

Fig. 61 Pyoderma gangrenosum. This lesion initially looks like a boil or infected follicle. As it spreads, undermining and destroying the surrounding dermis, the underlying soft tissues are exposed. Occurring in about 5% of people with ulcerative colitis, pyoderma generally responds to high-dose corticosteroid therapy. Colectomy is rarely needed to control this condition although it is effective.

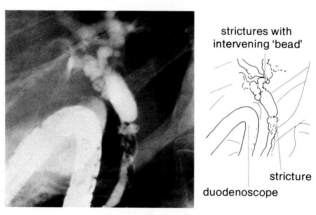

strictures with
intervening 'bead'

stricture

duodenoscope

Fig. 62 Sclerosing cholangitis. Most commonly seen as a complication of ulcerative colitis, sclerosing cholangitis produces a bead-like appearance due to numerous partial or complete biliary strictures with varying degrees of dilatation between. It is seen particularly where the main hepatic ducts meet. Biliary obstruction gradually develops but the progress of the biliary disease, which may produce secondary biliary cirrhosis, is independent of the activity of the ulcerative colitis.

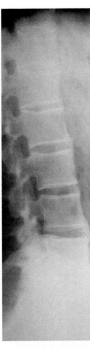 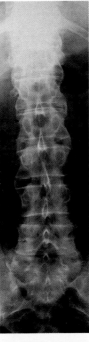

Fig. 63 Ankylosing spondylitis. The bony fusion of adjacent vertebrae can be clearly seen. Ankylosing spondylitis occurs 10 to 20 times more often in people with ulcerative colitis and Crohn's colitis than in the normal population. Spinal problems may occur before inflammatory bowel disease and their progression is independent of the activity of the latter. It is generally found more frequently in men but when associated with inflammatory bowel disease it occurs more commonly in women.

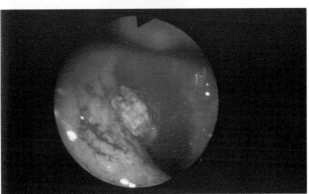

Fig. 64 Polyp in ulcerative colitis. An adenomatous polyp with surrounding mucosal inflammation. This patient had suffered from ulcerative colitis for nearly 20 years. On histological examination, the mucosa of the polyp was severely dysplastic amounting to carcinoma *in situ*. Similar mucosal abnormality was found elsewhere and a colectomy was performed. The incidence of carcinoma in ulcerative colitis is increased, particularly if the patient has total colitis, by a long disease duration (10 to 20 years) and by onset in youth.

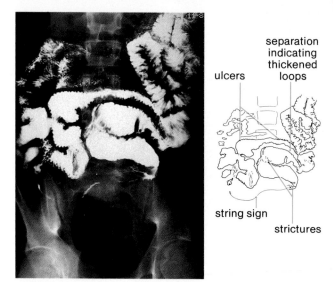

separation
indicating
thickened
loops

ulcers

string sign

strictures

Fig. 65 Crohn's disease of the ileum. The terminal ileum shows a long stricture, the string sign. The ileum proximal to this has several dilated loops with intervening strictures. Separation of the ileal loops is wider than usual, indicating mucosal disease and many deep ulcers are present.

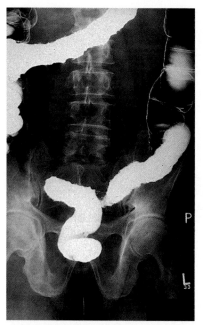

Fig. 66 Crohn's disease of the colon. This barium enema shows dilatation and ulceration of the transverse and sigmoid colon with a normal descending colon. These skip lesions with intervening normal mucosa are characteristic features of Crohn's disease. The ulcers in the sigmoid are deeper than those seen in ulcerative colitis.

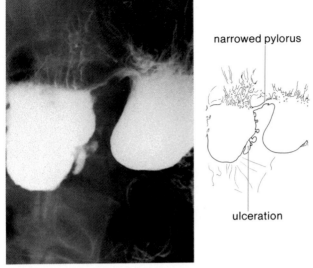

narrowed pylorus

ulceration

Fig. 67 Gastroduodenal Crohn's disease. It must be remembered that any part of the whole gastrointestinal tract is potentially the site of Crohn's disease. This radiograph shows a narrowed pylorus and ulceration in the adjacent duodenum.

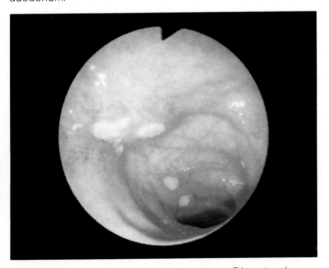

Fig. 68 Crohn's disease: aphthous ulcers. Discrete ulcers in the intestine with normal intervening mucosa is one of the typical features of Crohn's disease. They appear on the barium enema as small target lesions with a central pit and surrounding halo.

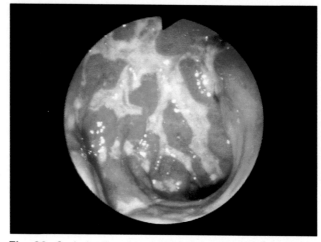

Fig. 69 Crohn's disease: cobblestoning. Extensive linear ulceration in the colon is seen interspersed with areas of inflamed oedematous mucosa. This produces the cobblestone pattern seen on barium studies. Over time and perhaps with treatment these lesions can heal as strictured areas or even revert to normal.

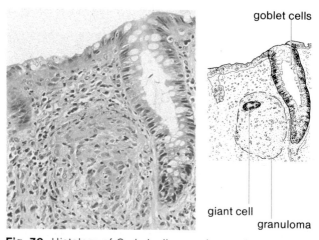

Fig. 70 Histology of Crohn's disease. A granuloma is present in the centre of the field. The cluster of pink epithelioid cells contains a giant cell. Although the mucosa is inflamed, the surrounding glands are relatively normal in appearance with numerous goblet cells. This finding in a biopsy from a rectum that appears normal is of great help in making a diagnosis of Crohn's disease. It also shows that Crohn's disease can have a patchy distribution micro-scopically as well as macroscopically. H & E stain.

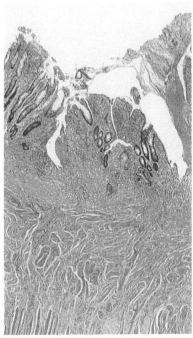

Fig. 71 Histology of Crohn's disease. This case is much more severe than that in Fig. 70. The mucosa shows discontinuous loss of glands; some of those which do remain look near normal. There are three deep fissure-like ulcers and the inflammation is not confined to the mucosa and submucosa but involves all layers of the intestine. Lymphoid aggregates are present. H & E stain.

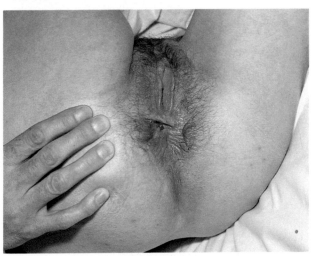

Fig. 72 Perianal Crohn's disease. Recurrent fistulation and its treatment have resulted in a distorted perianal region with prolapsing inflamed mucosa. Typical skin tags are also visible. Anal disease can occur in conjunction with small intestinal disease but without colonic involvement.

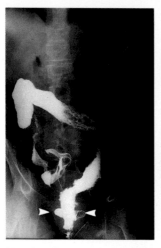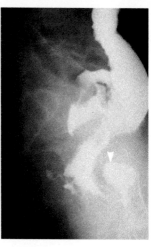

Fig. 73 Crohn's disease: rectovaginal fistula. This is a complication of Crohn's disease that is very rarely encountered in ulcerative colitis. Symptoms vary between patients but a slight vaginal discharge is the commonest. Faeculent material or flatus is passed much less frequently. The radiographs show vaginal filling as pouches (arrowed) on either side of the rectum on the posterior-anterior view and inside the curve of the inflamed rectum on the lateral view.

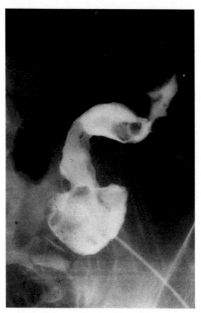

Fig. 74 Entero-cutaneous fistula. This fistulogram shows a catheter introduced into a cavity via the abdominal wall. As well as showing the cavity, contrast has entered the sigmoid colon which has a deep ulcer. This fistula was particularly indolent, discharging intermittently for over two years despite many different treatments. Entero-enteral fistulae are also commonly found in Crohn's disease.

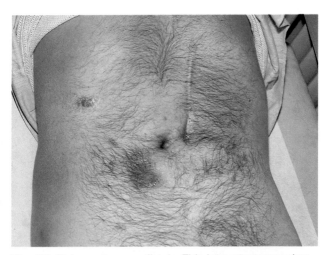

Fig. 75 Enterocutaneous fistula. This laparotomy scar has the opening of an intestinal fistula at the end adjacent to the umbilicus. The other purple areas that resemble healing fistulae are due to a resolving skin infection. Enterocutaneous fistulae in Crohn's disease, probably small intestinal in this instance, may need azathioprine or an elemental diet as initial therapy, with surgery being considered if medical management fails.

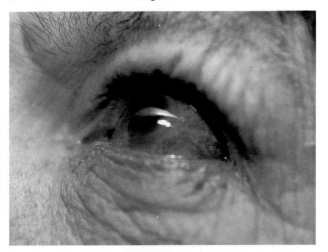

Fig. 76 Iritis. Iritis is a complication developing in about 5% of patients with ulcerative colitis and Crohn's disease. It is not related to the severity of the inflammatory bowel disease, only one third of cases being associated with an acute exacerbation. Other ocular lesions include episcleritis and keratitis.

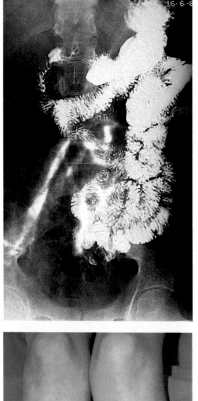

Fig. 77 Sacroiliitis. About 15% of patients with inflammatory bowel disease have sacroiliitis which may be found before the symptoms of stiffness and lower back pain develop. The right sacroiliac joint in this barium follow-through shows the abnormalities of sacroiliitis; a widened joint space and adjacent sclerosis are evident. A second complication of inflammatory bowel disease is an acute mono-arthritis that generally affects the large joints of the lower limb.

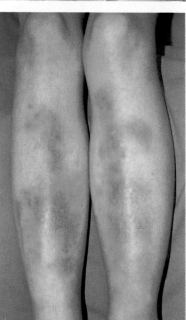

Fig. 78 Erythema nodosum. This is perhaps the most common cutaneous complication of ulcerative colitis and Crohn's disease. The lesions begin as red, raised, tender lumps, typically over the shin; they later change to purple and then yellow, fading over several weeks. Other vasculitic lesions may also be seen in inflammatory bowel disease.

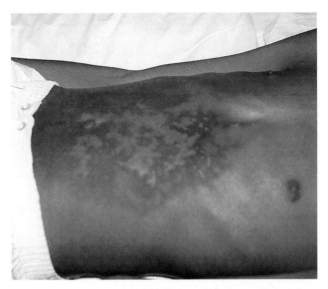

Fig. 79 Erythema ab igne. Heat, generally from a hot water bottle, frequently helps in abdominal pain. The severity and duration of this teenager's abdominal pain can be judged by the extent of the hot water bottle burns. He needed a resection of a strictured terminal ileum.

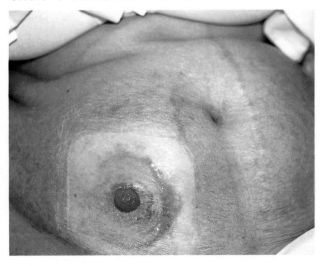

Fig. 80 Ileostomy. Ileostomies, formed following colectomy for inflammatory bowel disease or familial polyposis coli, are usually placed in the right lower quadrant. Gallstones and renal stones are more frequent in patients with an ileostomy and a cholecystectomy scar is also visible in this case.

42

DISORDERS OF THE LARGE INTESTINE

Those gastrointestinal diseases found in the Western World and not in the Third World are mostly large intestinal and are considered to be the result of the great dietary differences in these disparate communities. The most important disease with regard to morbidity and mortality is colonic carcinoma, the incidence of which is increasing. The most common is diverticular disease now found in many, if not most, elderly people. Intestinal parasites, and to a lesser extent tuberculosis, are major worldwide problems seen with varying frequency in Britain. As international travel increases these treatable disorders are being found more often. As the population becomes progressively aged, ischaemia is likely to be more common, the large intestine being the commonest site.

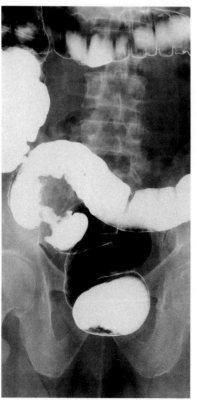

Fig. 81 Colonic carcinoma. A typical 'apple-core' lesion with an irregular outline is present in the sigmoid colon. The symptoms are usually an alteration in bowel habit with rectal bleeding. A carcinoma like this may be palpable. The differential diagnosis prior to barium enema includes diverticular disease, which may have identical symptoms. Carcinoma is a frequent cause of large intestinal obstruction in the elderly.

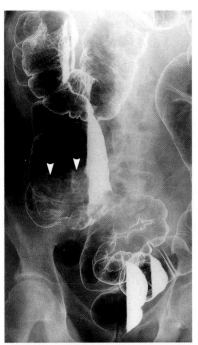

Fig. 82 Carcinoma of the caecum. Caecal carcinoma produces intestinal obstruction late in the course of the disease. This example (arrowed) is relatively large yet there was no obstruction to retrograde filling of the ileum and no dilatation of the small intestine. Symptoms may be those of anaemia or dyspepsia and weight loss reminiscent of benign or malignant gastric ulceration.

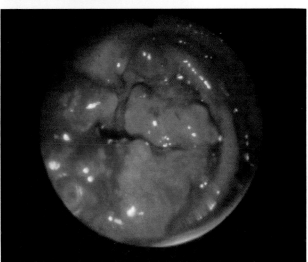

Fig. 83 Colonic carcinoma. This endoscopic view shows a typical colonic carcinoma filling the intestinal lumen with irregular masses of tumour. Histology is a useful prerequisite to surgery.

44

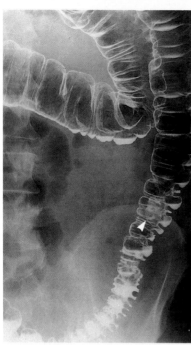

Fig. 84 Colonic polyp. In the middle of the descending colon lies a slightly irregular polyp (arrowed), about 2cm in diameter, on a stalk of a similar length. Diverticular disease is also present. Polyps, like carcinoma, are found most frequently in the rectum, sigmoid and descending colon. Bleeding, either occult or overt, is the commonest presentation.

The chance of a polyp being malignant increases with size, being under 2% if the polyp is less than 1cm in diameter, but 46% if over 2cm.

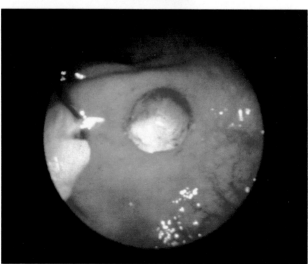

Fig. 85 Colonic polyp. A polyp is present on the colonic mucosa. Polyps of this size are often missed on a barium enema, particularly if complete clearance of faecal material can not be obtained.

45

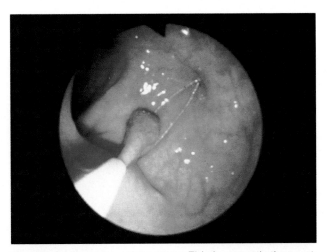

Fig. 86 Endoscopic polypectomy. This is currently the most common method used to remove polyps. The white outer sheath of the snare rests against the stalk of the polyp. The loop of the snare can be seen resting on the mucosa. The loop will be gradually tightened around the stalk until it is firm and a diathermy current can be used to excise the polyp which is then retrieved for histology.

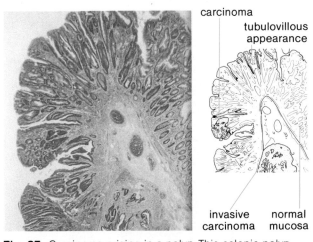

carcinoma

tubulovillous appearance

invasive carcinoma

normal mucosa

Fig. 87 Carcinoma arising in a polyp. This colonic polyp, removed endoscopically, shows several important features. The apex has the appearance of a tubulovillous adenoma. However, midway down the left side is an area of much more atypical mucosa amounting to carcinoma. The stalk has a triangular cross-section and contains invasive carcinoma. Adjacent normal mucosa is just visible on the right side of the polyp. H & E stain.

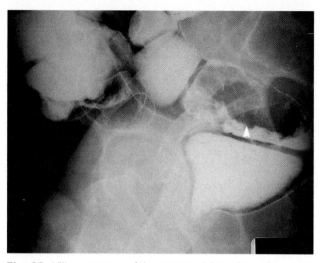

Fig. 88 Villous tumour of the rectum. A broad rectal tumour (arrowed) is seen arising posteriorly. Histological examination showed this to be a villous adenoma. A tumour of this size has a high probability of being malignant and it is too large and broad-based for endoscopic removal. Likely symptoms include the diarrhoeal passage of copious watery mucus, bleeding and tenesmus.

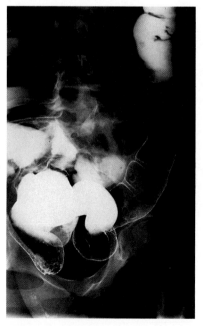

Fig. 89 Familial polyposis coli. This young woman's barium enema shows several polyps in the descending colon. Close examination of the rectum revealed numerous small polyps. Several members of her family had had a colectomy for polyposis coli. She underwent the same operation since carcinoma invariably develops in the untreated patient.

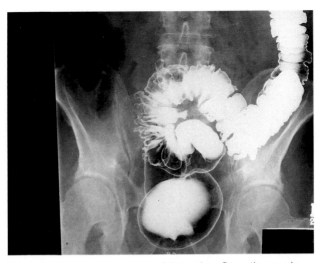

Fig. 90 Diverticular disease of the colon. Smooth muscle hypertrophy is thought to be an early event with a subsequent increase in luminal pressure and then out-pouching of the mucosa to produce the diverticula. These events are most frequently found in the sigmoid colon and result in the characteristic saw-tooth appearance of diverticular disease.

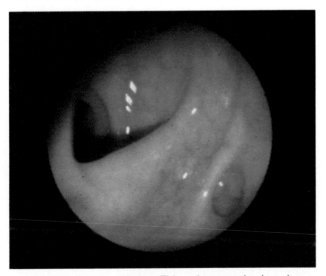

Fig. 91 Diverticular disease. This colonoscopic view shows the opening of a diverticulum as well as several prominent muscular folds. The mucosa generally looks normal, as in this patient, overt inflammation being rarely encountered.

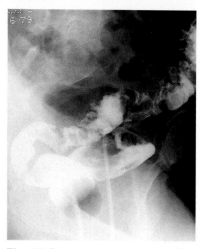
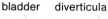
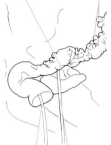

bladder diverticula

catheter catheter
in rectum in bladder

Fig. 92 Rectovesical fistula complicating diverticular disease. A barium-filled catheter has outlined the large intestine posteriorly, revealing numerous diverticula and saw-tooth haustrations. The bladder and a urinary catheter are filled with barium anteriorly. Frequency and pneumaturia are likely to expose the fistula but not the primary pathology. This results from diverticulitis, where a diverticulum has become an abscess draining into both the colon and the adherent bladder.

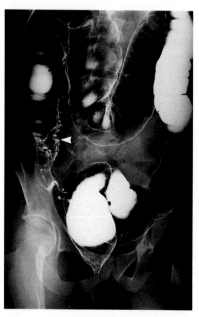

Fig. 93 Tuberculosis. Ileocaecal tuberculosis (arrowed) shares the radiological features of Crohn's disease from which it can be exceptionally difficult to distinguish. Formerly common, it is now mostly seen in Asian immigrants to Britain, in whom pulmonary tuberculosis is often apparent. Culturing the organism or histological proof are often needed to reduce the differential diagnosis.

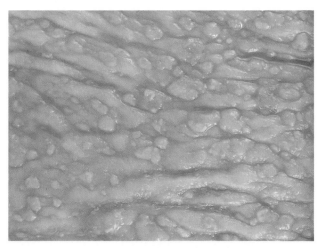

Fig. 94 Pseudomembranous colitis. An uncommon but potentially fatal result of antibiotic treatment, pseudo-membranous colitis presents as diarrhoea. The mucosa may be covered with small, yellowish, adherent plaques of pathognomonic histology. The administration of antibiotics has allowed *Clostridium difficile* to overgrow and both the organism and its toxin can be detected in the diarrhoea. Oral vancomycin or metronidazole are the current specific treatments.

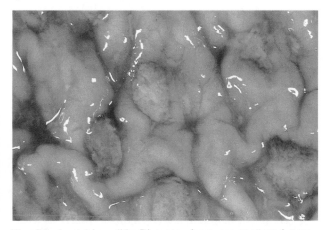

Fig. 95 Amoebic colitis. Discrete ulcers are scattered over the colonic mucosa. There is little surrounding inflammation but blood is present between the mucosal folds. There is a gradation in symptoms from the asymptomatic carrier state to fulminant colitis with profuse, bloody diarrhoea. Diagnosis is made by finding *Entamoeba histolytica* trophozooites in stools or rectal scrapes. Treatment is with metronidazole.

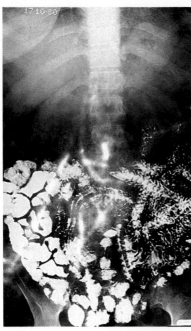

Fig. 96 Ascaris. Several roundworms are present in the small intestine. Barium can also be seen filling the intestine of a worm. Abdominal pain, either colic or diffuse, is the most common symptom. Heavy infestation with this worm, which is very common in the tropics, can produce intestinal obstruction or malabsorption.

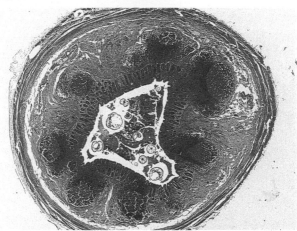

Fig. 97 Threadworms. In this appendix lie several threadworms, *Enterobius vermicularis*. Any family with symptomatic small children will know how troublesome they can be. Nocturnal pruritus ani with glimpses of the worms at the anal margin are recounted. Ova can be found on the perianal skin by day. As the ova are readily passed from person to person, the whole family should be treated twice, with a two week interval, to relieve the problem.

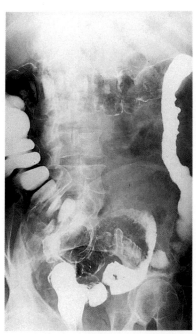

Fig. 98 Ischaemic colitis. The descending colon shows a narrow length of bowel with mucosal irregularity medially and ulceration and distortion laterally ('thumb-printing'). Healing can lead to a stricture in many of the patients who do not require an emergency laparotomy. Endoscopically, in an acute episode the mucosa is inflamed and ulcerated; it proves visually indistinguishable from inflammatory bowel disease.

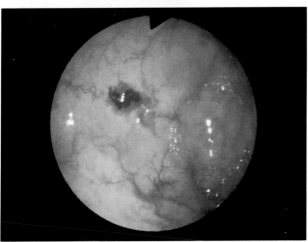

Fig. 99 Angiodysplasia. The cherry-red vascular malformation of angiodysplasia is evident and the surrounding vessels look slightly abnormal. Commonly found in the right colon, angiodysplasia can produce troublesome chronic bleeding but will not be visible on barium studies. Good bowel preparation before colonoscopy enables it to be seen and it can often be treated endoscopically.

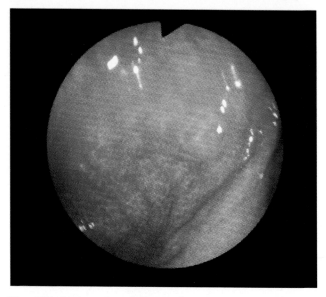

Fig. 100 Melanosis coli. Generally a consequence of prolonged laxative usage, this condition is manifest by brown pigmentation. Pale streaks are commonly seen dividing the darker areas into islands.

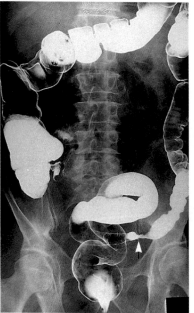

Fig. 101 Irradiation colitis. This stricture (arrowed) of the sigmoid colon was caused by irradiation. The intestines are sensitive to radiotherapy and great care is taken to minimise the exposure they receive. Diffuse bleeding can be troublesome in addition to the mechanical problems one would expect from the stricturing. Unfortunately, there is a high morbidity attached to surgical attempts to relieve these distressing problems.

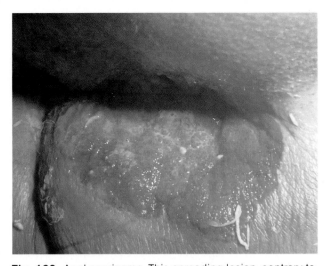

Fig. 102 Anal carcinoma. This spreading lesion, contrary to its appearance, is a squamous carcinoma and is often incorrectly diagnosed initially. Symptoms include pain and bleeding, or pruritus. Biopsy is very important whenever suspicions about perianal lesions are aroused. Management depends on the size and spread of the carcinoma.

PANCREATIC AND BILIARY DISORDERS

The pancreas lies deep in the upper abdomen and although the symptoms of pancreatic disease are often distinct it has been difficult to investigate until recently. Ultrasound, computer tomography and endoscopic retrograde cholangiopancreatography (ERCP) have revolutionised imaging of the pancreas. Nonetheless, chronic pancreatic disease remains a difficult and disheartening group of ailments to manage. Pain may be difficult to eradicate, alcohol abuse is important in some diagnoses and the prognosis of malignancy is appalling. On the other hand, the treatment of biliary disease is more rewarding for the clinician. Diagnostic approaches have advanced, as have therapeutic opportunities. Endoscopic therapy, percutaneous radiological intervention and gallstone dissolving techniques have helped many patients and hold considerable promise for the future. There are still many indications for surgery but fewer and fewer operations will be undertaken without a diagnosis and a specific purpose.

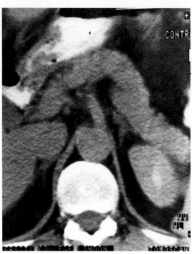

superior mesenteric artery

duodenum

pancreas

liver

spleen

aorta

left kidney

Fig. 103 Normal pancreas. The pancreas is seen arching across the field. The head, to the right of the patient, is adjacent to the liver and behind a contrast filled duodenum. The aorta, with the superior mesenteric artery arising from it, lies behind the pancreas. The tail of the gland overlies the left kidney and abuts the hilum of the spleen, just visible on the patient's left.

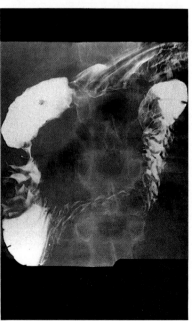

Fig. 104 Enlarged pancreatic head in acute pancreatitis. The duodenal loop is greatly widened, indicating an enlarged head of pancreas. This may be the result of acute or chronic pancreatitis or pancreatic carcinoma. The history with supporting investigations will give the diagnosis. Typical pain and a greatly elevated plasma amylase were features in this instance.

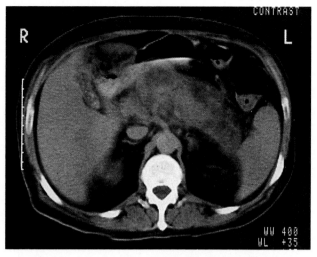

Fig. 105 Acute pancreatitis. Diffuse swelling of the pancreas with an indistinct outline are features of acute pancreatitis. Contrast is present in the duodenum between the pancreas and the liver. Gallstones and alcohol are the commonest causes, the former an indication for cholecystectomy and possibly some form of bile duct drainage.

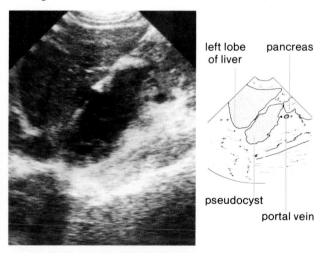

left lobe
of liver

pancreas

pseudocyst

portal vein

Fig. 106 Pancreatic pseudocyst. This complication should be suspected when abdominal pain and vomiting persist after an attack of acute pancreatitis. The plasma amylase remains elevated and an epigastric mass may be palpable. Small cysts resolve spontaneously but large cysts in the lesser sac generally require drainage into the stomach.

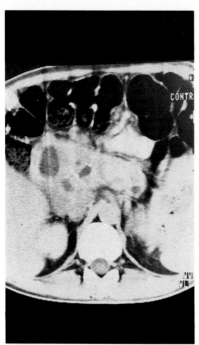

Fig. 107 Cysts in the pancreas. Several cysts are seen in this gland, the largest being in the head. They develop most commonly after acute pancreatitis and much less frequently in chronic pancreatitis. The new imaging techniques have demonstrated cysts much more often; instead of the 5-25% previously found, over 50% of cases have now been shown to have this complication. Cysts this size need follow-up, surgery being indicated only rarely.

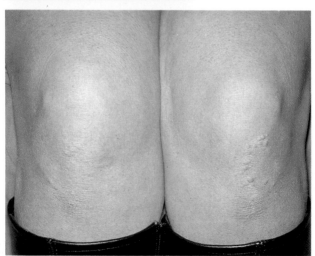

Fig. 108 Eruptive xanthomata. These eruptive xanthomata on the knees are due to hyperlipidaemia which may also cause recurrent attacks of pancreatitis. Other causes of pancreatitis, some remedial, include hereditary abnormalities, hyperparathyroidism and drugs.

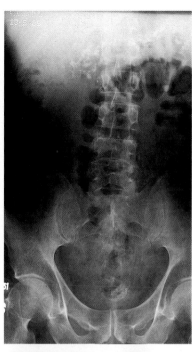

Fig. 109 Pancreatic calcification. Extensive calcification clearly outlines the pancreas, showing the head, the body lying over the first lumbar vertebra and the tail. Calcification typically occurs in chronic pancreatitis, being most frequent in, but not limited to, alcoholic pancreatitis. It is also detectable by the other imaging techniques used for the pancreas.

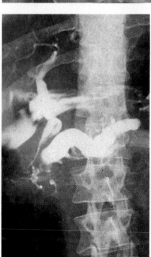

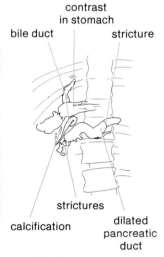

Fig. 110 Alcoholic chronic pancreatitis. Scattered calcification can just be seen in the head of the gland. The main duct is dilated and strictured. A smoothly tapering stricture of the bile duct due to extrinsic compression is present. A history of heavy drinking was obtained.

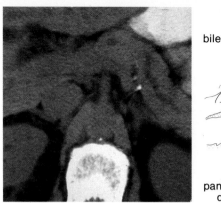
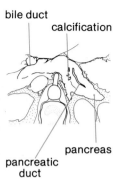

Fig. 111 Chronic pancreatitis. The pancreas is swollen on this CT scan and the dilated pancreatic duct can be clearly seen in the body and tail. Some calcification is present in the body and the bile duct is also dilated. Chronic, in common with acute pancreatitis, is most often related to alcohol or gallstones, although other rarer causes are recognised. The severity of the pain can lead to opiate addiction and malabsorption, malnutrition and diabetes mellitus add to the difficulties of management.

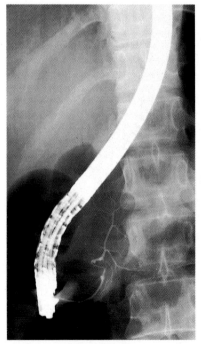

Fig. 112 Pancreas divisum. The main pancreatic duct has been filled but it is small and the duct system is greatly reduced. In pancreas divisum the dorsal and ventral buds of the pancreas fail to fuse fully during development, each retaining its own duct system. The body and tail drain through the accessory duct (not filled) and arise in the dorsal bud. Although uncommon, pancreas divisum is thought to be complicated by an increased incidence of symptomatic pancreatitis if there is narrowing of the accessory duct.

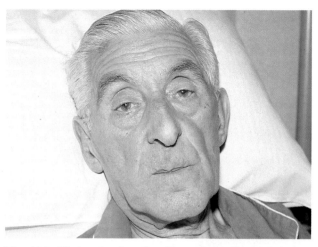

Fig. 113 Obstructive jaundice. The yellow sclerae of jaundice are evident in this patient. Obstructive jaundice is generally caused by gallstones or malignant disease. The former may be suspected with a history of indigestion, biliary colic or even rigors due to ascending cholangitis, and the latter if weight loss, abdominal pain radiating to the back and vomiting have occurred.

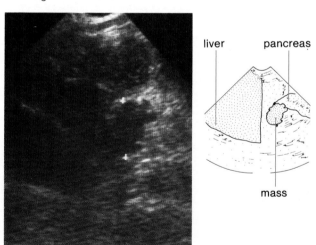

Fig. 114 Pancreatic mass causing obstructive jaundice. In this ultrasound a mass is present in the head of the pancreas. The pancreatic duct was found to be dilated indicating obstruction to both duct systems. Pancreatitis or pancreatic neoplasm could produce this appearance: an accurate history, appropriate biochemistry and even a guided aspiration cytology may be needed to reach a diagnosis.

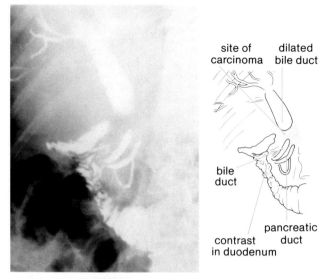

site of carcinoma dilated bile duct

dilated bile duct

bile duct

contrast in duodenum

pancreatic duct

Fig. 115 Pancreatic carcinoma. A carcinoma has completely obstructed the pancreatic duct and partially blocked the bile duct. Although the biliary stricture can not be clearly seen, the dilated proximal duct has filled. This patient had gnawing abdominal and back pain and then became jaundiced.

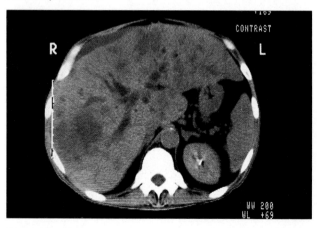

Fig. 116 Dilated bile ducts and metastases from pancreatic carcinoma. This enlarged liver appears abnormal with dilated bile ducts centrally which are in agreement with the patient's jaundice. Widespread metastases are present more peripherally. Other cuts showed a mass in the head of the pancreas and the diagnosis was subsequently confirmed histologically.

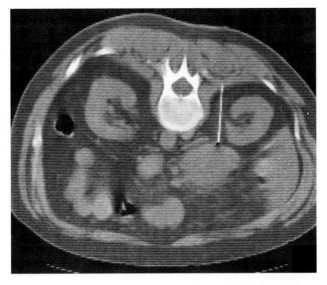

Fig. 117 Pancreatic carcinoma: aspiration cytology. A mass can be seen in the head of the pancreas. The patient is lying on his front so that aspiration cytology of the mass can be carried out. The CT has been used to guide the needle into the mass between kidney and spine.

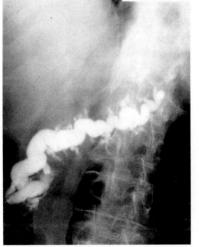

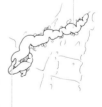

pancreatic duct

bile duct

Fig. 118 Periampullary carcinoma. A dilated obstructed pancreatic duct and partially filled dilated bile duct are visible. The gallbladder is palpable in 30% of these cases with painless jaundice. The operation of choice would be a Whipple procedure if there was no evidence of metastasis.

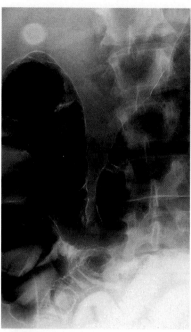

Fig. 119 Gall-
stones. In patients
with unexplained
abdominal pain, the
finding of a gallstone
which is calcified
(calcification
occuring in only 10%
of stones) can
provide a diagnosis.
This barium enema
demonstrates the
cause of vague
abdominal pain and
altered bowel habit
(due to dietary
changes) which was
cured when the
round, calcified
gallstone was
removed by a
cholecystectomy.

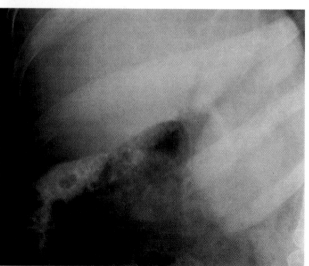

Fig. 120 Gallstones. The numerous large and small filling
defects seen on this cholecystogram are gallstones. During
an oral cholecystogram a fatty meal is given to stimulate
contraction of the gallbladder and, if successful, this often
makes the stones more apparent.

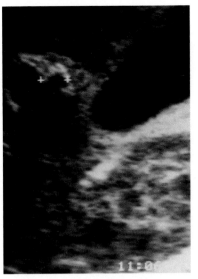
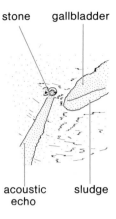

stone   gallbladder

acoustic   sludge
echo

Fig. 121 Gallstone. This ultrasound shows a gallstone in the neck of the gallbladder. The acoustic echo of the stone is clearly seen as well as the contents of the gallbladder with a layer of biliary sludge.

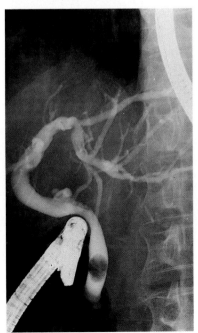

Fig. 122 Gallstone in the common bile duct. On this ERCP a filling defect in the bile duct is due to a gallstone. The patient had previously had a cholecystectomy. Sphincterotomy with an attempt at endoscopic stone extraction would be the next stage of the treatment. If this fails then a follow-up examination after an interval may show that the stone has passed spontaneously.

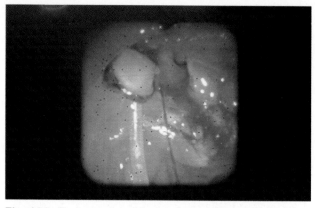

Fig. 123 Endoscopic sphincterotomy. A fragment of gallstone is seen emerging from the bile duct into the duodenum. The papilla of Vater has been opened by electrocautery using the wire which can be seen here with its sheath. Various baskets and balloons can be used to further clear the bile duct.

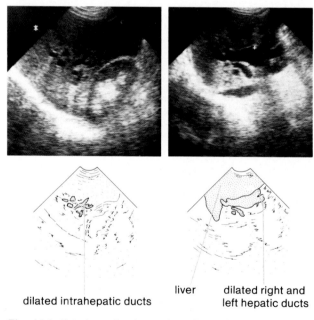

dilated intrahepatic ducts

liver   dilated right and left hepatic ducts

Fig. 124 Extrahepatic obstruction of the bile duct. Corkscrewing, dilated intrahepatic ducts (left) and a widely dilated (1.9cm) common hepatic duct (right) are visible. This was due to obstruction of the common hepatic duct, tumour being confirmed at subsequent laparotomy.

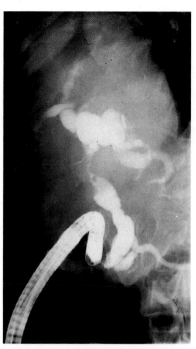

Fig. 125 Malignant stricture of the bile duct. A malignant stricture has caused considerable dilatation of the bile duct in this patient with obstructive jaundice. Only half of these patients have gallstones, unlike carcinoma of the gallbladder where stones are present in over 80% of cases. The failure to demonstrate the gallbladder in this instance may be due to malignant involvement of the cystic duct.

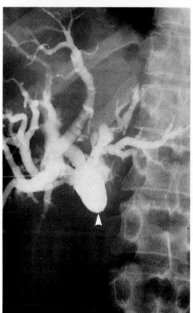

Fig. 126 Malignant stricture of the bile duct. This has been demonstrated by a percutaneous transhepatic cholangiogram (PTC). The fine needle used can be seen. It is advanced into the liver until bile is aspirated and then the biliary system can be filled with contrast. A blockage of the common hepatic duct (arrowed) is shown with no contrast entering the common bile duct.

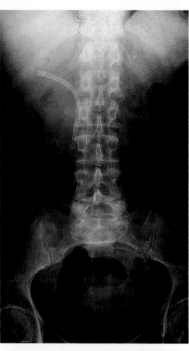

Fig. 127 Biliary prosthesis. Obstructive jaundice from pancreatic or bile duct carcinoma has a very poor prognosis and surgery is generally palliative at best. An alternative approach to the relief of jaundice has been the positioning of a prosthesis across the stricture. One end lies in the common hepatic duct and the other.in the duodenum. These prostheses can be introduced via an endoscope or percutaneously down the dilated biliary tree.

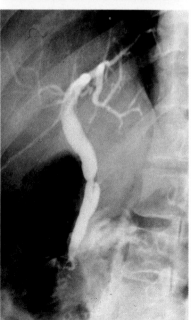

Fig. 128 Benign stricture of the bile duct. A benign stricture of the mid-portion of the bile duct is likely to be the consequence of damage at the time of cholecystectomy. The cystic duct enters the sheath of the bile duct at this level.

DISORDERS OF THE LIVER

The many functions of the liver in metabolism, detoxification and as a recipient of portal blood explain the diverse nature of the manifestations of liver disease. Worldwide, infections with hepatitis viruses, parasites and primary cancer are major problems of public health. In the Western World cirrhosis is becoming increasingly common. Particular problems associated with liver disease are the assessment of hepatic function when other treatment is planned and the care of the patient with decompensated cirrhosis. Many drugs are hepatotoxic and cause abnormalities of liver biochemistry in normal individuals. Their administration to patients with established liver disease can be extremely hazardous.

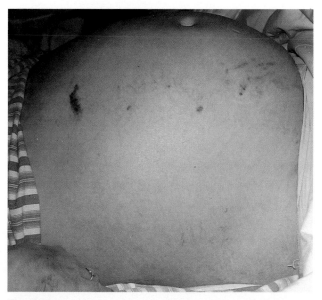

Fig. 129 Jaundice and ascites. This middle-aged alcoholic woman was admitted unwell. Ascites has produced distension of the abdomen and striae with bruising are also apparent. Ascites is best detected by shifting dullness. If only a small amount is suspected, both ultrasound and CT scanning will aid diagnosis. Diagnostic aspiration of ascites is important in determining its cause. Fluid can be drawn from the flank or the relatively avascular linea alba, as in this case. Jaundice is a common feature of acute alcoholic hepatitis, the cause in this patient.

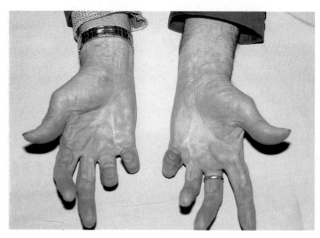

Fig. 130 Dupuytren's contractures. The palmar fascia is visibly and palpably thickened, being more pronounced when the little and ring fingers are extended fully. The contractures are most commonly found in alcoholic liver disease, although they are reported in cirrhosis due to other causes as well as in other non-hepatic diseases. This case is at an advanced stage with the fingers fixed in flexion. Previous surgical attempts to improve the function of the hand are apparent.

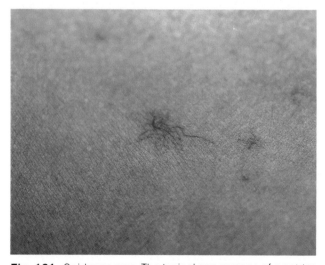

Fig. 131 Spider naevus. The typical appearance of a spider naevus is of a central feeding arteriole with radiating vessels. Pressure on the arteriole will blanch the whole naevus. Like Dupuytren's contractures, these naevi are most commonly seen in alcoholic patients but not exclusively so.

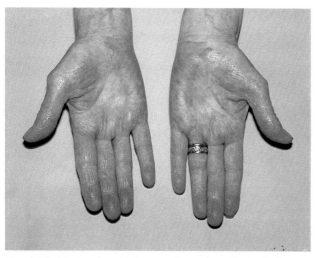

Fig. 132 Liver palms. Palmar erythema paradoxically leaves the centre of the palm pale compared to the redness of the surrounding thenar and hypothenar eminences and of the tissues over the metacarpophalangeal joints. It is important to look for other stigmata of liver disease as these changes are common.

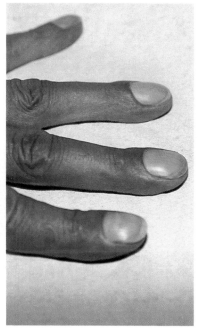

Fig. 133 Leuconychia and clubbing. Whitening of the nails and clubbing are both found in cirrhosis. This patient had cirrhosis due to hepatitis B positive chronic active hepatitis. Leuconychia is related to a low plasma albumin level, albeit poorly, and so may be seen in other hypoalbuminaemic states. Clubbing is also associated with other gastrointestinal disorders, particularly inflammatory bowel disease and coeliac disease.

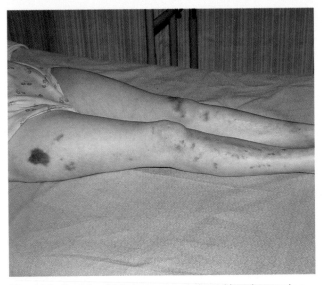

Fig. 134 Bruising. This is commonly found in advanced liver disease, particularly alcohol induced. It is likely to be caused by local trauma as well as a combination of prolonged clotting and a reduced platelet count.

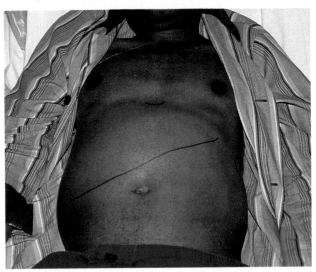

Fig. 135 Hepatosplenomegaly. Liver disease with portal hypertension is an important cause of hepatosplenomegaly. Haematological and tropical diseases are the other major causes of this finding. Other stigmata of liver disease may be found as well as abnormal liver function tests.

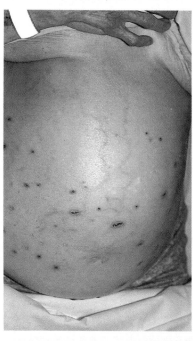

Fig. 136 Distended abdominal veins. Prominent abdominal veins can arise in portal hypertension. The remnant of the umbilical vein distends, acting as a collateral between portal and systemic venous sytems. Blood is then distributed into abdominal wall veins, the flow radiating out from the umbilicus. Alternatively, pressure on the inferior vena cava from ascites or tumour forces blood to flow through superficial low pressure veins. The flow will then be from pubis to chest.

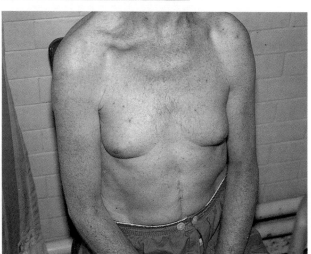

Fig. 137 Gynaecomastia. Gynaecomastia is a frequent finding in alcoholic cirrhosis and haemochromatosis but should be detected by palpation when just present. Gross gynaecomastia, as illustrated here, is generally found in association with testicular atrophy and absent body hair. The use of spironolactone to treat ascites increases breast size.

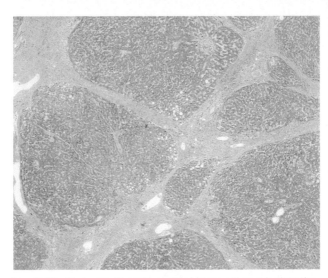

Fig. 138 Cirrhosis. Broad bands of fibrous tissue isolate the nodules of varying size. The liver cell plates, the arrangement of cells within the lobule, do not consist of uniform, one cell thick strands but are of variable size. It is important to remember that this histology may be found in a well person with no evidence for liver disease, i.e. well compensated cirrhosis.

	Group A good hepatic function	Group B moderate hepatic function	Group C poor hepatic function
Plasma bilirubin μmol/l	< 35	35–50	> 50
Plasma albumin g/l	> 35	35–30	< 30
Encephalopathy	none	minimal	advanced
Ascites	none	easily controlled	poorly controlled
Nutrition	excellent	good	poor

Fig. 139 Child's classification. The outcome of complications and their treatment in patients with cirrhosis depends upon hepatic function. An assessment of hepatic function can be made with Child's classification, patients in Group A having good function and low mortality whereas those in Group C include the 'end of the line' cirrhotic with a high mortality irrespective of any treatment attempted.

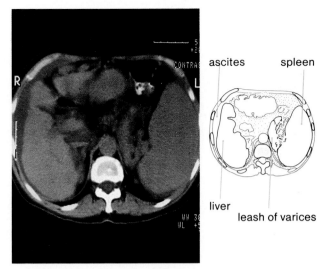

ascites   spleen

liver

leash of varices

Fig. 140 Cirrhosis and portal hypertension. The spleen is enlarged and a leash of varices is present at the splenic hilum. The liver is small and ascites is visible between liver and body wall, as well as elsewhere in the abdomen.

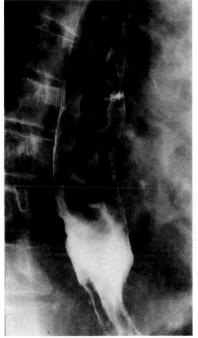

Fig. 141 Oeso-phageal varices and portal hypertension. The dilated submucosal veins have produced a tortuous impression in the column of barium in this case, but may be represented by irregularity and beading of the mucosa in other patients. They extend to the gastro-oesophageal junction. This patient's very large vessels were known to have ruptured on several occasions.

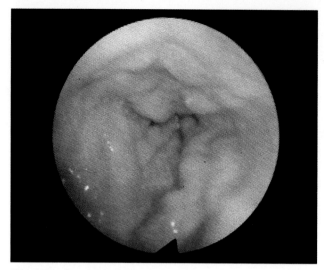

Fig. 142 Oesophageal varices. Serpiginous oesophageal varices can be seen snaking down the oesophagus. There are several cords of moderate size in this example. Purplish spots are often visible at the site of rupture if varices are the cause of haematemesis.

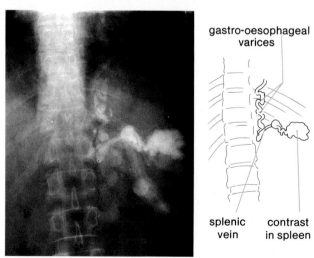

gastro-oesophageal
varices

splenic
vein

contrast
in spleen

Fig. 143 Splenoportogram of oesophageal varices. This technique involves injection of contrast medium into the spleen with sequential radiographs to follow its flow through the portal system and the collaterals. To the left of the spine are numerous dilated and tortuous veins which can be traced to the varices present above the diaphragm.

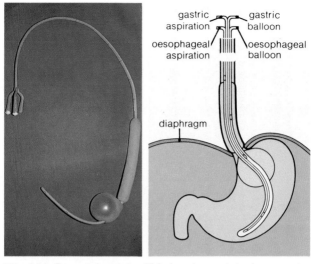

Fig. 144 Sengstaken tube. This four-lumen tube is passed into the stomach and the gastric balloon is inflated when over 40 cm from the teeth. Gentle traction will pull the balloon to the cardia where it will occlude varices. Inflation of the oesophageal balloon, with continuous pressure monitoring, may be needed. Aspiration of the upper oesophagus and stomach can continue through the two channels. Experience and skilled nursing are needed for its safe use.

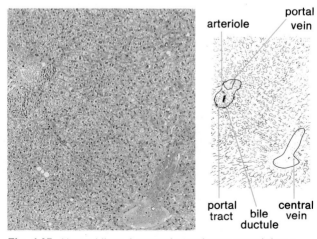

Fig. 145 Normal liver. A normal portal tract containing a portal vein, arteriole and bile ductule is demonstrated, as well as the centre of the lobule containing a central vein. The hepatocytes are arranged as cords between the two structures, each cord with liver cell plates only one cell thick.

Fig. 146 A comparison of chronic persistent and chronic active hepatitis. Histology is the ultimate method of classifying chronic hepatitis. Chronic persistent hepatitis follows viral infection. Chronic active hepatitis in Britain is most commonly autoimmune, then hepatitis B related, but may rarely be caused by Wilson's disease, alcohol and drugs including methyldopa.

	Chronic persistent hepatitis	Chronic active hepatitis: autoimmune	Chronic active hepatitis: hepatitis B associated
Symptoms	malaise, tiredness, fat and alcohol intolerance	malaise, anorexia, jaundice, joint pain, rashes, abdominal pain	malaise, poor recovery from hepatitis B
Predominant age and sex	all ages, both sexes	younger women	men over 30
Signs	hepatomegaly	hepatosplenomegaly, spider naevi, palmar erythema, jaundice, acne	hepatosplenomegaly
Associated illness	none	autoimmune disease including thyroid, ulcerative colitis, fibrosing alveolitis	glomerulonephritis, arthritis, polyarteritis nodosa
Outcome	good prognosis, no treatment needed	cirrhosis and death if not treated with corticosteroids, may progress rapidly	slow progression to cirrhosis or hepatoma, no effective treatment

77

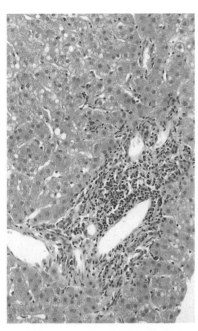

Fig. 147 Chronic persistent hepatitis. The portal tract near the edge of this needle biopsy contains a greatly increased number of inflammatory cells. The demarcation between the portal space and the liver substance, the limiting plate, is intact.

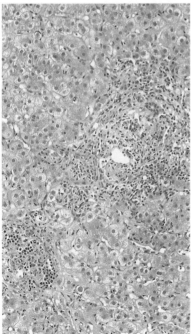

Fig. 148 Chronic active hepatitis. Two adjacent portal tracts are shown. Although both contain an excess of inflammatory cells the limiting plate does not confine changes and inflammation is spreading out like tentacles. Some hepatocytes have been surrounded and look abnormal (piecemeal necrosis). The inflammation is also linking the two portal tracts producing bridging necrosis and starting to separate the liver substance into nodules.

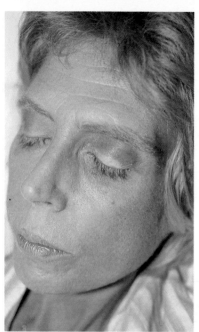

Fig. 149 Primary biliary cirrhosis. This middle-aged woman was deeply jaundiced at presentation, the pigmentation having taken two to three years to achieve this colour. Her plasma bilirubin was 450µmol/l . She also had pruritus, anorexia and recent weight loss. The xanthelasmata are especially prominent.

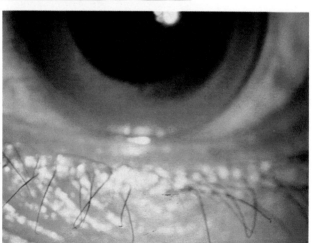

Fig. 150 Wilson's disease. Brown pigment has been deposited in the outermost cornea to form a Kayser-Fleischer ring. The liver is vulnerable to progressive accumulation of metals. The inherited conditions of Wilson's disease, due to copper accumulation, and haemochromatosis, due to iron accumulation, are good examples. Both progress to cirrhosis if untreated.

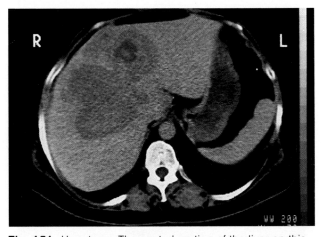

Fig. 151 Hepatoma. The central portion of the liver on this CT scan is replaced by a mass which shows necrosis in its most anterior part. Liver biopsy confirmed the diagnosis of hepatoma, which had extended to the diaphragm producing partial collapse of the right lower lobe and a small pleural effusion. Most hepatomas are found in patients with cirrhosis or chronic hepatitis B infection and there are great differences in incidence in different parts of the world, for example it is the commonest malignancy in Mozambique.

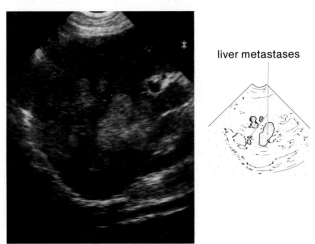

liver metastases

Fig. 152 Liver metastases. Numerous echo-dense metastases are present in the liver. Complaining of right upper quadrant abdominal pain and having abnormal liver function tests, this patient's metastases were confirmed by ultrasound. She had had a previous hemicolectomy for carcinoma.

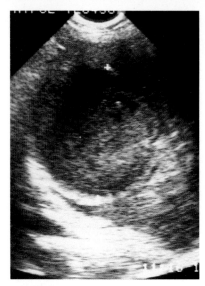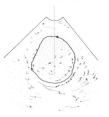

amoebic abscess

Fig. 153 Amoebic abscess. A large abscess cavity in the liver is shown in a patient who had a high fever and a painful, tender liver. The right diaphragm was elevated on chest X-ray. Reddish pus containing amoebae was aspirated and metronidazole used in treatment.

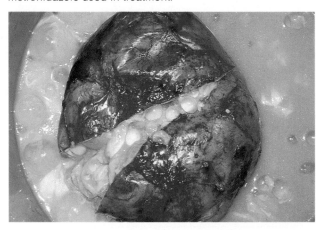

Fig. 154 Hydatid cysts. Rare in the British Isles, hydatid disease is not infrequently encountered in Eastern Europe and the Middle East. Symptoms, if any, include abdominal swelling and pain. When suspected, diagnosis should be made by non-invasive means as fatal anaphylaxis may result from leakage of cyst fluid. Careful surgery to remove the cysts intact, as shown here, is the preferred treatment, although some antihelminthic agents may be effective.

81

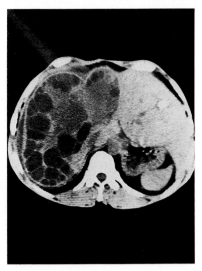

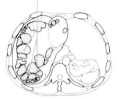

hydatid cysts

Fig. 155 Hydatid cysts in the liver. Numerous daughter cysts and the chitinous capsule can be readily seen. The left lobe of the liver is enlarged without obvious cysts, presumably due to compensatory hypertrophy.

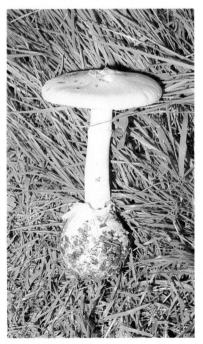

Fig. 156 Death cap (*Amanita phalloides*). Environmental causes of liver disease include carbon tetrachloride, phosphorus and iron as well as the most deadly fungal species known, the death cap, which produces hepatic and renal failure with 50-90% mortality. Drugs of many categories are a potent and frequent cause of hepatic dysfunction producing such syndromes as intrahepatic cholestasis (chlorpromazine), hepatitis (halothane), and hepatic necrosis (paracetamol overdose).

INDEX

abdomen, distended veins, 72

abscess, amoebic, in liver, 81

achalasia, 9

alcohol
and erosive gastritis, 16
and liver disorders, 68–72
and pancreatic disorders, 54, 56, 58

Amanita phalloides, 82

amoebic
abscess in liver, 81
colitis, 50

ampulla of Vater, carcinoma, 62

angular stomatitis, 23

ankylosing spondylitis, 34

anus
carcinoma, 54
Crohn's disease, 38

Ascaris, 51

ascites, 68, 72

aspirin, 4, 16

barium swallows, 1–7, 9–10
normal, 1

bile ducts
carcinoma, 62, 66
disorders of, 54, 58, 61–7
gallstones in, 64–5
prosthesis, 67
strictures of, 65–7

bladder, rectovesical fistula, 49

bleeding, gastrointestinal, 14–16, 20–1

bones, malabsorption and, 24

bowel disease, inflammatory, 27–42

bruising in liver disease, 71

caecum, carcinoma, 44

carcinoma
anus, 54
bile ducts, 62, 66
caecum, 44

colon, 43–4, 46
gallbladder, 66
oesophagus, 6–7, 10
pancreas, 60–2
stomach, 18–19
in ulcerative colitis, 34

Celestin tubes, 8

cholangitis, sclerosing, 33

coeliac disease, 23, 24, 25

colitis
amoebic, 50
Crohn's, 28, 35–40
irradiation, 53
ischaemic, 52
pseudomembranous, 50
ulcerative, 28–31
complications of, 32–4, 40–41

colon
angiodysplasia, 52
carcinoma, 43–4, 46
Crohn's disease, 35
disorders of, 43–54
diverticular disease, 48–9
melanosis coli, 53
parasites, 51
polyps, 45–7
toxic dilatation, 32
tuberculosis, 49

Crohn's disease, 28, 35–8
complications, 39–41
histology, 37–8

death cap, 82

dermatitis herpetiformis, 25

diverticular disease, 48–9

duodenitis, 14

duodenum
Crohn's disease, 36
disorders of, 11–14, 15
scars, 14
ulcers, 12–14, 15

Dupuytren's contractures, 69

dysphagia, 1
sideropaenic, 10

emepronium bromide, 4
enterocutaneous fistula, 39–40
enteroenteral fistula, 39
erythema ab igne, 42
erythema nodosum, 41
eyes, lesions in inflammatory bowel disease, 40

fingers, clubbing, 70
fistulae
  enterocutaneous, 39–40
  enteroenteral, 39
  rectovaginal, 39
  rectovesical, 49

gallbladder, carcinoma, 66
gallstones, 63–5
  and jaundice, 60
gastritis, erosive, 16
gynaecomastia, 72

haemochromatosis, 72, 79
haemorrhage, gastrointestinal, 14–16, 20–1
hands, signs of liver disease in, 69–70
heartburn, 1
hepatitis, chronic, 77–8
hepatoma, 80
hepatosplenomegaly, 71
hiatus hernia, 2–3, 5
hydatid cysts in liver, 81–2
hypertension, portal, 72, 74

ileostomy, 42
ileum, Crohn's disease, 35
indigestion, 1
intestines
  large *see* colon
  small
    blind loop syndrome, 26
    disorders of, 22–7
    diverticula, 26
    giardiasis, 27
    iritis, 40
iron deficiency, 23
irradiation colitis, 53

jaundice
  and ascites, 68
  cirrhosis and, 79
  obstructive, 60, 66–7
joints in inflammatory bowel disease, 41

koilonychia, 10, 23

leiomyoma, stomach, 19–20
leuconychia, 70
liver
  amoebic abscess, 81
  cirrhosis, 70, 72, 73–4, 79
  disorders of, 68–82
    drugs and, 82
    environmental causes, 82
    signs of, 69–72
  function, assessment of, 73
  hepatitis, 77–8
  hydatid cysts, 81–2
  metal accumulation and, 79
  normal, 76
  tumours, 80
Looser's zones, 24

malabsorption, 22–7
Mallory-Weiss tear, 16
melanosis coli, 53
monilial oesophagitis, 10
mouth
  angular stomatitis, 23
  ulcers, 32

naevus, spider, 69
nails
  koilonychia, 10, 23
  leuconychia, 70

odynophagia, 1
oesophageal varices, 74–6
oesophagitis
  monilial, 10
  reflux, 3
oesophagus
  achalasia, 9
  carcinoma, 6–7, 10
  disorders of, 1–10
  scleroderma, 9

spasm, 1
strictures
  benign, 4, 5–6, 9–10
  malignant, 4, 6–8
ulceration, 4
varices, 74–76
webs, 10
osteomalacia, 24

pancreas
  calcification, 58
  carcinoma, 60–2
  cysts, 57
  disorders of, 54–62
  divisum, 59
  normal, 55
  pseudocyst, 56
pancreatitis
  acute, 55–6
  causes, 56, 57
  chronic, 58–9
polyposis coli, 47
portal hypertension, 72, 74
potassium, slow-release, 4
primary biliary cirrhosis, 79
pseudofractures, 24
pseudopolyps, ulcerative
  colitis, 29–31
pylorus, stenosis, 17
pyoderma gangrenosum, 33

rectovaginal fistula, 39
rectovesical fistula, 49
rectum, tumours, 47
roundworms, 51

sacroiliitis, 41
scleroderma, oesophagus, 9
Sengstaken tube, 76
sideropaenic dysphagia, 10
spider naevus, 69
spondylitis, ankylosing, 34
stomach
  carcinoma, 18–19
  Crohn's disease, 36
  disorders of, 11–21
  erosions, 16
  leiomyoma, 19–20
  ulcers, 11–12, 14–15

telangiectasia, hereditary
  haemorrhagic, 20–1
threadworms, 51
tuberculosis, ileocaecal, 49

ulcers
  aphthous, 32
  duodenal, 12–14, 15
  gastric, 11–12, 14–15
  mouth, 32
  oesophagus, 4
  peptic, 11–15
    perforated, 17
  stomal, 21
  see also colitis

vagina, rectovaginal fistula,
  39
varices, oesophageal, 74–76
veins, abdominal,
  distension of, 72
vitamin deficiency, 23

Whipple's disease, 26
Wilson's disease, 79

xanthomata, eruptive, 57